MODERN MEDIC
IS MAKING US SICK!

Synthetic drugs, X-rays, surgery, etc., are sources of stress. Disease, aging, and nervous disorders are the results of stress. Is it any wonder that today we are substituting new illnesses for old sicknesses?

What can help us resist the ravages of stress without producing harmful side effects? For thousands of years, the people of eastern Asia have used ginseng, a natural remedy that comes from the root of a wild forest herb.

Until recently, modern authorities would not take its therapeutic properties seriously. However, with the recent emphasis on the natural environment, and the opening of communication between East and West, there appears to be a meeting of the modern scientific mind and traditional wisdom bred of an ancient culture. Science is regarding the products of nature with new interest. As research continues, there are indications that nature may have provided what the laboratory could not.

The Book of Ginseng presents this evidence in understandable terminology. A definitive survey of a subject that, for centuries, has fascinated scientist and layman alike!

THE BOOK OF
GINSENG

Sarah Harriman

▲PYRAMID BOOKS • NEW YORK

THE BOOK OF GINSENG

A PYRAMID BOOK

Third printing May, 1974

ISBN 0-515-02988-2

Library of Congress Catalog Card Number: 74-4596

Copyright © 1973 by Sarah Harriman

All Rights Reserved

Printed in the United States of America

Pyramid Books are published by Pyramid Communications, Inc. Its trademarks, consisting of the word "Pyramid" and the portrayal of a pyramid, are registered in the United States Patent Office.

PYRAMID COMMUNICATIONS, INC.
919 Third Avenue
New York, New York 10022, U.S.A.

To Jerry

Contents

Preface

The late sixties and early seventies have witnessed a groundswell of reevaluation of social and cultural patterns in the Western World. The most notable controversies have arisen from new awareness of the similarity of all people everywhere, despite surface differences. This awareness has stimulated a growing demand for equality—in the home, in the community, in the country, and in the world at large. Our new-found consciousness of the worth of others allows us to try things that might formerly have been dismissed simply because they were foreign.

A spirit of questioning has invaded the land, a spirit reflected in the ecology movement and the vastly increased interest in natural foods and natural lifestyles. Many people no longer believe that progress is the *raison d'être* of civilization. Dissatisfied with the quality of life offered by conventional modes, they seek alternatives.

This book is written to encourage the popular mood toward questioning and experimentation. While focusing on the solar system and its minute counterpart, the atom, in search for the secrets of life, perhaps we should at the same time ignore political divisiveness and share the knowledge accumulated by earthbound civilizations more ancient than our own.

1

Herbal Wisdom of the Ancients

Dr. E. Grey Dimond, director of The Cardio-
vascular Center in Kansas City, Missouri, made
an investigatory trip to mainland China. On his
return he stated that he "expected herbal reme-
dies would follow acupuncture as the next medic-
inal import from China."

—THE NEW YORK TIMES,
September 13, 1972, p. 17

WESTERN MEDICINE has long considered the folk medicine of Asian peoples to be of little consequence
when compared with the efficacy of modern "miracle
drugs." But perhaps the value of ancient remedies
should be reconsidered. Unable to cure many diseases
with synthetic drugs and disturbed at the decline in
general health brought about by modern lifestyles,
many physicians feel that natural medicines may indeed hold secrets of health and longevity.

For thousands of years Oriental peoples have depended largely on natural herbal remedies—even today China and Korea rely on "barefoot doctors" to
provide medical service to the vast areas still not
reached by modern facilities. Through trial and error
a remarkable body of folk knowledge became established over the centuries—knowledge passed down
through the generations to the present day. Can the
faith of so many millions of people be dismissed without investigation? Dr. Dimond observes, ". . . There is
a tremendous amount of useful information in tradi-

tional herb medicine. The further I look into it, the more impressed I become. This is not a cult, not a 'lady with tea leaves'—they have had four thousand years of a pragmatic human laboratory."

The traditional Chinese viewpoint considers man to be one with nature, contrary to the man-over-nature concept prevalent in the West. Man is seen as insignificant within the vast scope of the natural world. Consider the typical landscape paintings of the Chinese, which often show the tiny figure of a traveler or seeker greatly overshadowed by towering cliffs or an expansive, gentle vista.

Chinese medicine teaches that human life in all its phases is inextricably interwoven with all other life forms. The causes of health and disease are directly related to imbalance of the forces of the universe. As Edward H. Hume describes this principle:

> There are life-preserving and life-destroying forces everywhere, acting alike on man and on plants and animals. It is the concern of medicine to neutralize the malevolent influences of the environment by the help of friendly spirits, to bring to man's aid every friendly force in nature, and to use, for the patient's restoration, medicaments that have not only what the West calls pharmacological value, but that are also, in themselves, akin to the forces of life and vigor.[1]

Yin and Yang

Five thousand years ago the great Chinese philosopher Lao-tzu used the word *tao* to describe the laws of the natural universe, the Eternal Way:

> Something there is,
> Whose veiled creation was
> Before the earth or sky began to be;

So silent, so aloof, and so alone,
It changes not, nor fails,
But touches all:
Conceive it as the mother of the world.
I do not know its name;
A name for it is "Way."

Tao-te Ching

Thus the "Way" means the natural way of things, the order of nature. *Tao* is eternal, unchangeable, all-pervasive, unity, indescribable, nameless. The Taoist principle underlies the concepts fundamental to Chinese medicine. In the beginning, it is believed, order was created out of Chaos when the Great Absolute (*T'ai Chi*) separated to form the metaphysical and the material principles. The positive, metaphysical Yang and the negative, material Yin together constitute the Cosmos. Harmonious balance between the cosmic forces of Yin and Yang contribute to order within the universe and health within the body of man. Yin is considered passive and feminine, comprising the weaker phenomena of cold, darkness, expansion, and so on. Yang is considered active and masculine, comprising the stronger phenomena of heat, light, constriction, and so forth. Yin and Yang are direct opposites, but at the same time they are complementary. No object or organism is ever completely Yin or completely Yang.

Based on the cosmic principle of Yin-Yang interaction, the philosophy of Chinese medicine evolved an elaborate system of relationships. Without this fundamental philosophy Oriental medicine cannot exist, contrary to modern medicine, which has generated its own *raison d'être*. Chinese philosophy as it relates to medicine is described in detail elsewhere.[2] It is sufficient to quote here the *I Ching*:

When Heaven and Earth exert their influence all things are transformed and vivified.

Ancient Origins of Herbal Knowledge

The oldest surviving body of medical knowledge reputedly is that of the Chinese. Exact dates are difficult to establish, for writers of ancient times were known to attribute their works to still more ancient sources, probably to enhance the value of their observations. The boundaries between fact and legend have become obscured by time; nevertheless, it is certain that Chinese medicine is rooted in the very soil that gave rise to Chinese civilization.

Among the foremost cultural heroes of China is the Emperor Shen-nung, who traditionally is said to have lived from 3737 to 2697 B.C. To Shen-nung is attributed the founding of agriculture and the first experiments with herbal remedies. The legendary emperor was conveniently blessed with a transparent covering across his abdomen, through which he could observe the inner working of his body and note the effects of various herbal remedies. He compounded and self-tested hundreds of herbal preparations. His observations were preserved in the first pharmacopoeia, called the *Pen-ts'ao,* or *Herbal.* The *Pen-ts'ao* lists 365 preparations and their medical applications. The majority of these medicaments are herbal in nature; of the rest, forty contain animal material and eleven contain minerals.

In its legendary antiquity, the *Pen-ts'ao* is rivaled only by the *Huang-ti Nei-ching,* the *Yellow Emperor's Classic of Internal Medicine.* Huang-ti, the Yellow Emperor (traditional dates, 2697-2595 B.C.), was a primal ancestor with mythological standing equal to that of Shen-nung. The *Nei-ching* is written in the form of a dialogue between Huang-ti and his chief minister, Ch'i Po. It discusses general principles of health and presents a comprehensive treatment of anatomy and physiology. The cosmic forces that determine health and disease are stressed, as are methods of diagnosis and the principles of acupuncture.

Anachronisms in both the *Pen-ts'ao* and the *Nei-ching* indicate that they were written long after their mythological dates would have it—probably late in the first millennium before Christ. Nonetheless these works are based on the empirical knowledge gained from experimentation over the course of many centuries. The use of herbs to alleviate disease probably was common long before the beginnings of agrarian culture.[3]

The *Nei-ching* was followed by several pharmacopoeias written by eminent Chinese physicians. The most definitive of these works is the *Pen-ts'ao Kang-mu*, a distillation of the therapeutic knowledge of the ages compiled by the physician Li Shih-chen near the end of the sixteenth century A.D. Li Shih-chen presents the natural remedies of Chinese medicine in a most meticulous way, listing more than 1,800 medicinal preparations. To the medicaments of the ancients he added his own special formulations. The result is a pharmacopoeia still much consulted by folk doctors in modern China.

Materia Medica

The Chinese draw on a vast number of sources when devising remedies. The *Pen-ts'ao Kang-mu* alone lists 492 medicaments of animal origin; 1,094 medicaments of vegetable origin (610 herbs, 484 trees and shrubs); 275 medicaments derived from metals and minerals; and 31 "everyday articles."[4]

These substances generally are not thought to "cure" in the modern Western sense of prophylaxis and the immune reaction. Rather, Chinese folk remedies seek to maintain or reestablish within the body the balance of cosmic forces, without which health and vigor are unobtainable. Much of Chinese medicine is directed at *maintenance* of health. Prevention is the honored function of the physician, and it is said that the people once paid their physician as long as they were healthy, but he paid them if they became ill. In the words of the poet Shao Tze, "It is better to avert a malady with care than to use a physic after it has appeared."

Some of the animal constituents of Oriental remedies are repellent to the Western mind. Certain remedies contain, for example, crushed centipedes, powdered rhinoceros horn, mouse excrement, human skullbone, dragon's blood, or the urine of a young boy. But to the Oriental mind, no thing that is a product of nature is an object of distaste. Of course, a great deal of superstition attends the popularity of these remedies, and belief may be nine-tenths of the cure in some cases. A Chinese proverb observes, "When you treat disease, first treat the mind."

Probably more reliable are the remedies of herbal and mineral origin. Indeed, many mighty weapons of modern medicine were discovered in the folk remedies of various cultures. Among the modern drugs originally obtained from plants long used by folk doctors are these:

Iodine, originally derived from seaweed by Polynesians for use externally as a fungicide and bactericide.

Digitalis, extracted from foxglove (*Digitalis purpurea*); first used by an English folk doctor and employed today in congestive heart failure.

Reserpine, derived from *Rauwolfia serpentina*, now

used to treat essential hypertension and certain neuropsychiatric disorders; long used by Hindus as a tranquilizer.

Penicillin, a powerful antibacterial substance obtained from the bread mold *Penicillium;* first discovered by Greek shepherds, who applied the mold to heal wounds.

Rhubarb, the dried root and rhizome of *Rheum officinale,* used as a cathartic; first used in China 5,000 years ago.

Ephedrine, isolated from the plant *Ephedra sinica,* called *ma huang* in China; acts as a decongestant; chemically synthesized ephedrine is widely used today.

Cannabis, the dried flowering tops of Indian hemp or marijuana, long used in India as a pain reliever, hypnotic, and antispasmodic; sometimes prescribed in the West as a sedative.

Quinine, a specific for malaria, yielded by *Cinchona* bark; first used by Jesuits in Peru.

Castor oil, from the castor-bean plant *Ricinus communis,* acts as a cathartic; first used 2,000 years ago in India as a purgative.

Opium, yielded by the opium poppy *(Papaver somnifer),* produces the narcotic analgesics morphine and codeine and the muscle relaxant papaverine.

Camphor, Cinnamomun camphora, long used in the Far East for its antiseptic and anesthetic properties.

All these drugs were scorned by physicians until careful experimentation proved the value of the plant remedies. How many other effective natural remedies await the endorsement that can come only through meticulous application of the scientific method? The pharmaceutical organizations of every advanced country in the world yearly expend vast sums in trying to answer that very question.

Panacea from the Forest Floor

Among the most honored remedies included in Oriental pharmacopoeias is one derived from a rather

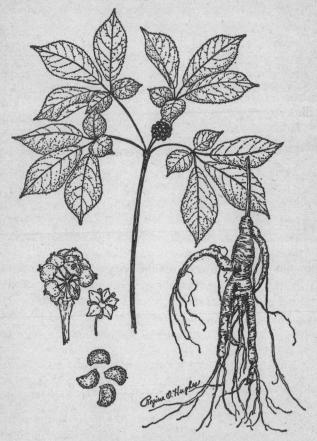

Branch, root, flower, berries, and seeds of American ginseng.

unprepossessing plant called *ginseng,* which grows sparsely in mountainous woodlands in certain parts of Asia. Its taxonomic name, *Panax ginseng,* stresses its fabled curative and restorative properties (*Panax,* from the Greek word meaning "all-healing") and the fancied resemblance of its root to the human body (*ginseng,* from the Chinese words *shen seng,* meaning "man-root").

The medicinal properties of ginseng are attributed to substances contained in the root. Extracts of ginseng are believed by the Chinese—and, as we shall see, by many other peoples—to have both generally healthful effects and specific action against certain disorders of the human body.

Panax ginseng is native to China, Korea, and Siberia. Its North American counterpart, *Panax quinquefolium* ("five-fingered root".), is also believed to have medicinal value and appears in the medicinal folklore of many American Indian tribes. Both species are classified in the botanical family Araliaceae. They are elusive plants of dense forest and have very exacting requirements for cultivation. Their scarcity lends extremely high value to a root of fine quality.

The plant is a low, perennial shrub bearing three to five compound leaves on a single stalk and sending up a single cluster of flowers each spring. The root is creamy or white and resembles a parsnip with rootlets branching off to suggest the shape of the human body (see Chapter 7).

Extracts of ginseng, ginseng tea, and the root itself have a peculiar sweetness, accompanied by bitter undertones. There is little or no odor. The bulk of the root is starchy and contains small amounts of resin, volatile oil, and *panaquilon,* which is the medicinally active substance of the root.

A related plant, *Eleutherococcus senticosus,* indig-

enous to Siberia, has properties similar to those of
ginseng and is being investigated in laboratories
across the USSR to extract its medicinal secrets.

All varieties of ginseng have become the subject of
intensive experimentation, documented in Chapter 6,
as scientists seek to explain the faith of the Chinese in
their panacea, ginseng. Perhaps ginseng, long over-
looked by modern science, will at last be given everywhere the position of importance it has held in the
Orient for centuries.

2

The Root of Heaven

WHITNEY ROBERTSON is an energetic West Coast industrialist who at the age of sixty-three has the
physique and vigor of a much younger man. He eats
well but sparingly, runs six to ten miles a day, and
chews a bit of ginseng root every morning and eve-
ning. An aura of brimming vitality surrounds him, and
his young companion enthusiastically attributes her
good fortune to the ginseng. Mr. Robertson is one of
many Westerners who have discovered the healing and
revitalizing properties of ginseng, the parsniplike root
fabled as a medicinal magician in the Orient.

Traditionally, the Chinese claim ginseng to be

". . . a tonic to the five viscera, quieting animal spirits,
establishing the soul, allaying fear, expelling evil
effluvia, brightening the eye, opening up the heart,
benefiting the understanding, and if taken for some
time it will invigorate the body and prolong life."[1]

The *Pen-ts'ao Kang Mu*, still in use among Chinese

doctors, attributes to ginseng the properties of an alterative, tonic, stimulant, carminative, and demulcent. All of which means that ginseng is thought to rebuild tissues, give tone to the body, stimulate energy, ease gripping pains and expel flatulence, and soothe and protect the alimentary canal. Ginseng is prescribed by folk doctors both to strengthen and revitalize persons weakened by disease and to increase the vigor of healthy persons. It is thought to have a cumulative effect as a tonic—ginseng each day keeps the doctor away. Its general effect is to rejuvenate the body and strengthen it against the debilitating effects of stress, both mental and physical.

The Herb of Eternal Life

Does ginseng prolong life? Many Eastern people believe so; indeed, ginseng is widely supposed to be the "herb of eternal life" referred to in ancient legend. As a tonic, it is possible that ginseng could have some beneficial effect in warding off the symptoms of senescence. But it must be noted that in the Orient the elderly are respected for their experience and wisdom. Unlike Western peoples, who shun the approach of old age and its discomforts, Eastern people tend to welcome old age as a time for reflection and basking in the wealth of love and regard showered on them by their respectful families.

There is some evidence that the climacteric—the physical and mental changes accompanying the transition from middle age to old age—does not occur in the same way among all cultures. The Navaho, for example, view old age not as a time of waning physical and sexual capacities, but as a time of grace and increased personal importance. As Sol Worth, professor of visual communications at the University of Pennsylvania, observes:

At age forty-five, when all most of us [Americans] have to look forward to is getting knocked off, the Navaho is stepping into a new hierarchy. Now he is a leader. He doesn't have to perform. His children and grandchildren can ride the horses and climb the mountains and be virile. He does other things better, like giving advice. ... Climacteric depression as a biocultural event doesn't appear to exist here.[2]

This observation applies equally to the Chinese: The real Oriental fountain of youth probably is cultural rather than medicinal. Nevertheless, as a strengthener of the central nervous system (brain and spinal cord) and a regulator of blood pressure, ginseng taken regularly may help prevent two of the major problems of old age—senility and high blood pressure. Jeannie Rose, in her marvelous compendium of things herbal, describes the rejuvenating regimen of a Chinese herbalist named Li Chung Yun: He drank a daily tea of ginseng and fo-ti-tieng (*Hydrocotyle asiatica minor*); ate only those vegetables that grow above ground; drank only mineral water; and maintained a serene attitude at all times.[3] According to records kept by the Chinese government, Li Chung Yun lived to be 256 years old (1677-1933).

Aphrodisia

Like the industrialist described at the beginning of this chapter, many people believe that ginseng acts as an aphrodisiac and maintains sexual potency in the human male. The origin of this idea probably lies in the primitive pattern of thought commonly called the "doctrine of signatures," which held that nature places a "sign" on certain plants to indicate their medicinal value. Thus lungwort (*Lobaria pulmonaria*), a plant that resembles the spongy surface of a human lung, was used to treat tuberculosis, pneumonia, and similar ailments in ancient Greece. Similarly, because the root of ginseng resembles the human body, it gained a reputation of having power in matters procreational. In fact, ginseng does stimulate the formation of healthy cells in both male and female reproductive organs (and elsewhere in the body) and so may encourage successful procreation.

Ginseng is considered the most Yang (masculine in action) of all herbs. True believers have been known to wear a well-shaped root as a sexual amulet, and it is said that a Chinese emperor once paid $10,000 for a particularly shapely man-figure root. Among wealthy Oriental aristocrats the very best grades of ginseng formerly commanded considerable respect and high prices, for it was valued as an aid in keeping concubines satisfied. Ginseng was—and still is—taken by a man before intercourse to enhance his performance, and perhaps after a strenuous sexual encounter to rebuild his sapped energy and restore potency.

According to a classic of Indian knowledge, the *Atharva-Veda*, ginseng

> . . . aids in bringing forth seed that is poured into the female that forsooth is the way to bring forth a son. . . . The strength of the horse, the mule, the goat, and the ram, moreover, the strength of the bull [ginseng] bestows on him. . . . This herb will make thee so full of lusty strength that thou shalt, when thou art excited, exhale heat as a thing on fire.[4]

Paul Kourennoff reports that ginseng causes gray hair to regain its color and the wrinkles of age to vanish. Unconfirmed tales of aged men siring children abound in China and Korea, where "ancient Casano-

vas boast openly of their sex prowess and attribute
this to the use of ginseng."[5]

By contributing to general health and vigor, ginseng may well enhance a man's virility and sexual in-
clinations. After chewing ginseng root or sipping an
extract of the herb, the user is washed with a wave of
pleasant warmth and invigoration. What better state
of body and mind exists in preparation for love-mak-
ing? Of course, the most effective aphrodisiac will always be a case of mind over matter. As John Lilly has
observed, "In the province of the mind what one be-
lieves to be true either is true or becomes true."

Ginseng as an aphrodisiac has its adherents in the
West, too. The proprietor of a New York health food
store volunteered, "Man, the stuff really turns me
on—one dose and I'm there!" When I asked for
ginseng extract in another health food emporium, the
clerk pushed a bottle across the counter, leered rather
shyly, and muttered, "Is good for the sex, eh?"

Tonic Nature of Ginseng

Dr. Lin Yutang, who was born in China and earned
a master's degree at Harvard University and his doc-
torate at Leipzig, has spent his life as a lecturer and
writer about China. This urbane devotee of ginseng
praises "the magic tonic and building qualities of ginseng, for which I am willing to give personal testi-
mony; it is the most enduring and most energy-giving
tonic known to mankind, distinguished by the
slowness and gentleness of its action."[6]

The Chinese describe cases in which a sick man almost at the point of death has been sufficiently re-
vived by a dose of ginseng to transact final items of
business.

The use of ginseng as a tonic is a daily matter—one
chews a bit of root or takes a spoonful of extract each

morning on an empty stomach. Taken alone, ginseng gradually and gently encourages the body to gain vigor and resilience. This strengthening effect accounts for the widespread belief in ginseng as a panacea. Of all the tests to which modern scientists have subjected ginseng, not one has shown even the slightest deleterious side effect of this herb. Considering that even so innocuous a synthetic drug as aspirin has been shown to have dangerous side effects under certain conditions, perhaps it is time for modern science to reevaluate this most gentle "queen of the herbs."

Preparation of Ginseng Tonic

Ginseng extract is made by decocting the root in water and evaporating the solution as described in this traditional Korean formula:

Take ten ounces of ginseng, cut it into small slices, put it to infuse in twenty small porcelain vessels of spring or river water till it is thoroughly soaked, and then pour the whole into a stone or silver vessel. Boil the infusion over a gentle fire made of mulberry wood until half the water is wasted. Then, having strained off the juice, pour ten middling porcelain vessels upon the solid matter; let this solution boil until it is reduced by half. To the remaining liquid add five cups of water to the ten vessels that you previously strained off; boil it over a gentle fire until it is of syrupy consistency.[7]

The extract produced by this recipe must be kept in a tightly closed container. Note that no metal should ever come in contact with ginseng, with the exception of silver.

The following updated recipe is easier to understand and should produce similar results: Soak overnight one ounce of sliced ginseng root in two cups of water in a covered glass bowl. The next day, simmer the root and water together in an enameled pan, covered, over a very low flame for two or three hours. Cool, and strain the liquid into a glass container with a tight-fitting lid. If you wish, chew the remaining solid matter to be sure you haven't missed any medicinal ingredients that might be left in the root.

Ginseng extract is used alone or in formulas of several ingredients, to which the ginseng contributes its tonic and constructive properties and enhances the potency of the other drugs contained in the remedy.

Most Chinese medicines are administered as a decoction or infusion of the ingredients, and many have traditional standing in medicinal folklore. In these concoctions certain herbs appear again and again in combination with ginseng—among them are ginger, licorice, fou ling, cassia, and huang ch'i. Ginger (Zingiber officinale) is a pungent and aromatic plant whose rhizome is used as a stimulant and to expel gas from the stomach and bowel. Licorice root (Glycyrrhiza glabra) is widely used in cough remedies and serves as a soothing emollient in preparations designed to treat conditions of the chest and lungs. Fou ling (Pachyma cocos) is an Asian herb believed to ease chest pains, invigorate the body, and prolong life. Cassia bark (Cinnamomum cassia), or Chinese cinnamon, yields a substance that acts as a tonic, soothes the stomach, and expels gas. Huang ch'i is a Chinese species of locoweed (Astragalus hoantschy), which acts to promote perspiration and stimulate internal warmth.

Examples of herbal formulas of the ancients are given in this chapter; they are culled from the Chinese Pen-ts'ao Kang-Mu, the Korean Pang-yak-hap-pyun, and other sources. Many of these recipes are still in use today in the Orient, but they are presented here only for their historical interest and are not intended as a guide to self-medication. Several of the herbs used medicinally in the Orient are native only to Asia and do not have English names. Many of the formulas are only general guides for the healer, who adapts them to the specific needs of his patient.

TONIC DECOCTION

(*Ssu-chun-tze-t'ang*)

For a tonic useful in all conditions of wasting and weakness, equal parts of the following ingredients are combined:

Ginseng extract
P'ai chu (*Atractylis ovata*)
Fou ling (*Pachyma cocos*)
Dried licorice root (*Glycyrrhiza glabra*)
Ginger (*Zingiber officinale*)
Dates (*Phoenix dactylifera*)

TINCTURE OF GINSENG

(*Jen-shen-chiu*)

Powder ginseng root and ferment it with rice and leaven (yeast), or digest powdered root in prepared spirit. Used as a tonic in all wasting diseases.

DATE AND GINSENG PILLS

(*Tsao-shen-wan*)

This preparation is made by pounding together ginseng root and large dates of Southern China. The pills are intended to strengthen the respiratory organs.

PURPLE CLAVARIA PILLS

These pills contain ginseng and sixteen other medicinal plants having tonic properties, all bound together with honey. The pills are said to be "a most wonderful tonic and reconstructive remedy in all wasting diseases."

CANTONESE TONIC

(*Sap-tsunn-tai-po*)

Prescribed for men and women who suffer from diminution of vital power, loss of appetite, occasional fever, weakness of the legs, laborious and strained breathing, jaundiced appearance, spermatorrhea (involuntary flow of semen without copulation), or weakness of the spleen or kidneys. This preparation strengthens both Yin and Yang principles simultaneously. It contains

Ginseng root	2 parts
Cassia bark (*Cinnamomum cassia*)	2 parts
Licorice root (*Glycyrrhiza glabra*)	2 parts
Root of Chinese white peony (*Paeonia albiflora*)	3 parts
Root of *huang ch'i*, a milkvetch (*Astragalus hoantschy*)	4 parts
Root of spikenard (*Aralia edulis*)	3 parts
Root of *Conioselinum univittatum* (a plant resembling angelica)	2 parts
Root of *Atractylis lancea*, a kind of thistle	3 parts
Fou ling (*Pachyma cocos*)	3 parts
Prepared root of *ti huang* (*Rehmannia glutinosa*)	4 parts

WHITE TIGER POTION

"For outer heat and inner coldness, dry palate, cold hands and feet, and general weakness of the body. Produces sweat and quenches thirst."

Chih mu (*Anemarrhena asphodeloides*)	6 liang
Powdered gypsum	1 chin
Licorice root (*Glycyrrhiza glabra*)	2 liang
Rice, ground (*Oriza sativa*)	6 liang
Ginseng extract	3 liang

(In Chinese measurement, 1 liang equals 1.33 ounces avoirdupois and 16 liang equals 1 chin, or 1½ pounds.)

Or, for similar symptoms, cook the following ingredients in 5 liters of water, boiling rapidly until the liquid is reduced to 2 liters:

Ginseng extract	3 liang
Ginger (*Zingiber officinale*)	3 liang
P'ai chu (*Atractylis ovata*)	3 liang

This preparation is to be drunk three times a day, one cup per dose.

GENERAL TONIC

A gentle tonic recommended for strengthening the spleen and the stomach; considered unsurpassed as a tonic for increasing Yang forces and increasing appetite. Sometimes prescribed for digestive troubles.

Ginseng extract	2 parts
Root of *Atractylis lancea*, a kind of thistle	2 parts
Fou ling (*Pachyma cocos*)	2 parts
Licorice root (*Glycyrrhiza glabra*)	1 part

TONIC FOR AGUE

For agues of various kinds, ginseng is recommended extensively in a series of prescriptions. The following formula is suggested for ague, characterized by alternating fever and chill:

> Root of *ch'ail hu* (*Bupleurum falcatum*) 2 mace
> Chinese white peony (*Paeonia albiflora*) 1 mace
> Licorice root (*Glycyrrhiza glabra*)   1 mace
> Ginger (*Zingiber officinale*)   3 slices
> Ginseng extract   1 mace
> *Pan-hsia* (*Pinellia ternata*)   1 mace
> Jujube (*Zizyphus vulgaris*)   two
> Cassia bark (*Cinnamomum cassia*)   1 mace

(In Chinese measurement, 1 mace equals 58½ grains.)

Ginseng as Panacea

Ginseng is prescribed by one source or another for treatment of many disease conditions of serious consequence. G. A. Stuart tells us that in China ginseng has for centuries been considered helpful in cures for debility, spermatorrhea, severe dyspepsia, chronic malaria, fevers of all kinds, exhausting discharges, chronic coughs, and polynuria.[8] A British customs official reported from China in 1884 that he found ginseng to be a "panacea par excellence," strengthening in cases of debility and also emetic in nature. In addition, Chamfrault and Ung Kang Sam[9] report that ginseng traditionally has been prescribed in remedies for

- tuberculosis
- fitful coughs
- nausea
- diabetes
- thirst accompanied by flushed skin and dry throat
- indigestion
- diarrhea
- dysentery
- degeneration of the kidneys, characterized by continual thirst, polyuria, and pain in the renal area (above small of back)
- enuresis
- gout
- rheumatism in the lower limbs
- suppurating sores

Remedies for some of these afflictions have more or less traditional standing in Chinese folk medicine; a sampling follows.

RESOLVENT DECOCTION

(*Chih-chung-t'ang*)

The following ingredients are combined in solution:

Ginseng extract
P'ai chu (*Atractylis ovata*)
Ginger (*Zingiber officinale*)
Licorice root (*Glycyrrhiza glabra*)

The preparation is used to reduce swellings produced in the course of any disease of the viscera, especially the heart, lungs, or spleen.

FUNGUS POWDER

(*Mu-chan-ssu-san*)

Powder together equal parts of

Fungus growth scraped from a camphor tree (*Cinnamomum camphora*)

Ginseng root

Whiteleaf Japanese magnolia (*Magnolia hypoleuca*)

Snake gourd (*Tricosanthes multiloba*)

Wild ginger—*hsi hsin* (*Asarum sieboldi*)

Siler (*Siler divaricatum*)

Ginger (*Zingiber officinale*)

Balloon flower—*chieh keng* (*Platycodon grandiflorum*)

Used to heal carbuncles and all sorts of cancerous and infected sores.

SEVEN PRECIOUS POWDER

(*Ch'i-pao-san*)

Powder together equal parts of

Dragon bone

Elephant's skin

Dragon's blood

Ginseng root

Gimura pinnatifida

Olibanum (frankincense—a resin from trees of the genus *Boswellia*)

Myrrh (*Commiphora myrrha*)

Laka wood

This preparation promotes healing of wounds and was a favorite among military men. One wonders when they found time to do battle, what with slaying dragons, gathering herbs and resins, and skinning elephants (presumably strays).

DIABETES REMEDY

A general tonic for daily use in cases of diabetes contains

Ginseng root	1 part
Root of milk vetch (*Astragalus hiroshimanus*)	3 parts
Root of spikenard (*Aralia edulis*)	3 parts
Root of *Atractylis lancea*, a kind of thistle	10 parts
Fou ling (*Pachyma cocos*)	3 parts
Root of *ti huang* (*Rehmannia glutinosa*)	10 parts
Fruit of Cornelian cherry (*Cornus officinalis*)	6 parts
Root of Japanese yam (*Dioscorea japonica*)	6 parts
Rhizome of water plantain (*Alisma plantago*)	3 parts
Root of tree peony—*mu tan* (*Paeonia moutan*)	3 parts
Skunk bugbane—*sheng ma* (*Cimicifuga foetida*)	1 part

The combined ingredients are formed into small pills.

INDIGESTION REMEDY

This medicament is used to ease indigestion following overeating, accompanied by upset stomach, heaviness, and constipation. All these symptoms characterize a weakness of the spleen, which this preparation purports to strengthen.

Ginseng extract	2 parts
Root of *Atractylis lancea,* a kind of thistle	2 parts
Peel of bitter orange (*Citrus aurantium*)	2 parts
Baelfruit (*Aegle sepiaria*)	2 parts
Fruit of Chinese hawthorn (*Crataegus pinnatifida*)	3 parts
Wheat germ	3 parts

TCHONG KING'S REMEDY FOR DIARRHEA

Considered useful for treatment of Yin diarrhea or Yin dysentery when the extremities are icy, perspiration is profuse, and the pulse is somewhat feeble and deep.

Root of wolfbane—*fu-tze* (*Aconitum fischeri*)	2 parts
Ginseng extract	2 parts
Rhizome of ginger (*Zingiber officinale*)	2 parts
Root of *Atractylis lancea,* a kind of thistle	2 parts
Licorice root (*Glycyrrhiza glabra*)	1 part

REMEDY FOR ENURESIS

In cases of involuntary urination, excessive urination, or urine that falls drop by drop at the end of urination, the following preparation is often suggested.

Fruit of Chinese magnoliavine— *wu-wei-tze* (*Schizandra chinensis*)	2 parts
Fruit of Cornelian cherry (*Cornus officinalis*)	3 parts
Ginseng root	3 parts

Seeds of cardamom
(*Elettaria cardamomum*)   3 parts

All the ingredients, except ginseng, are broiled in a frying pan with a little salt before combination.

REMEDY FOR INSOMNIA

For use as a sedative, the Chinese prepare a formula comprising equal parts of chopped ginseng, dried orange peel, and honey. Oddly enough, the stimulating properties of ginseng do not seem to provoke the nervous reactions typical of synthetic stimulants. Taken at bedtime, ginseng is soothing and calming.

REMEDY FOR LEPROSY

A prescription to be taken at the onset of leprosy consists of *pai-ch'ih* (a variety of angelica), crushed scorpions, and ginseng.

SEVEN FAIRIES POWDER

(*Ch'i-hsien-tan*)

Smallpox remedies abound in Oriental herbal medicine. The dread associated with this disease by all peoples is apparent in the "magical" ingredients included in many of the remedies devised specifically for smallpox. Seven Fairies Powder contains:

Milk vetch (*Astragalus hoantschy*)	2 ounces
Ginseng root	1 ounce
Licorice root (*Glycyrrhiza glabra*)	1 ounce
Truelove (*Paris polyphylla*)	1 ounce
Plum blossoms (*Prunus domestica*)	1.5 ounce
Monochasma savatieri	1 ounce
Human skullbone, powdered	1 piece

Ingredients are powdered together, then used to prevent smallpox or to modify the eruptions if smallpox has already taken hold.

TWO FLOWERS POWDER

(Erh-hua-san)

This preparation is used in treatment of smallpox. To any quantity of yellow plum blossoms or peach blossoms dried in the shade, the following powdered ingredients are added:

Hawthorn fruits (*Crataegus*), pitted and roasted
One small gourd (*Luffa cylindrica*), dried in the shade
Orange peel (*Citrus aurantium*)
Ginseng root
Milk vetch (*Astragalus hoantschy*)
Licorice root (*Glycyrrhiza glabra*)
Vermilion (a red pigment, mercuric sulfide)
Truelove (*Paris polyphylla*)
Monochasma savatieri
Scaly anteater
One human tooth
One piece of skull

GINSENG SMALLPOX REMEDY

(Jenn-chenn-ping-fey)

When cough accompanying smallpox is severe, the following preparation is often suggested:

Inner rind of Russian mulberry root
    (*Morus tartarica*)   4 grams
Root of *chih-mu* (*Anemarrhena*
    asphodeloides)   2 grams

Licorice root		
(*Glycyrrhiza glabra*	2 grams	
Rind of Chinese litchi nut		
(*Nephelium litchi*)	2 grams	
Mandarin orange peel		
(*Citrus reticulata*)	2 grams	
Fou ling (*Pachyma cocos*)	1 gram,	40 grains
Root of black hellebore		
(*Helleborus niger*)	1 gram,	40 grains
Ginseng root	1 gram,	40 grains
Chinese magnoliavine		
(*Schizandra chinensis*)		20 grains

Ingredients are to be powdered together and taken in an infusion of ginger (*Zingiber officinale*).

Pregnancy and Childbirth

Because of its strengthening properties, ginseng is often prescribed in Chinese medicine for pregnant women, both to ease discomforts and to strengthen the body before childbirth.

T'A CHING

It is suggested that for several days preceding the birth, the mother should drink a solution of the following herbs powdered together and dissolved in warm water:

Root of Chinese lovage	
(*Levisticum officinale*)	4 grams
Root of white peony	
(*Paeonia albiflora*)	4 grams
Root of *p'ai chu*	
(*Atractylis ovata*)	4 grams
Betelnut (*Areca catechu*)	4 grams

Mandarin orange rind (*Citrus nobilis*)	3 grams	
Crumbled leaves of sweet basil (*Ocimum basilicum*)	3 grams	
Ginseng root	3 grams	
Licorice root	1 gram	20 grains

If delivery is difficult, a little ginseng extract may be given after each contraction. If the woman is very weak after delivery, ginseng is given several times daily to hasten her recovery.

Tonics for Infants

Ginseng is considered beneficial to constitutionally frail children; a small bit of root or extract given daily will have a revitalizing effect.

A fever in a newborn child is a serious matter, and steps to counteract it must be taken quickly. Chinese medicine suggests two different remedies, *pao-long* and *kin-ting*. Both are made in pill form and one or two pills of either kind should be dissolved in a tea of ginger or mint. Both kinds of pills are to be rolled in gold leaf before use.

PAO-LONG

Yellow amber (fossil resin)	3 grams
Ginseng extract	3 grams
Sandalwood (*Santalum album*)	3 grams
Roasted licorice root (*Glycyrrhiza glabra*)	6 grams
Fou ling (*Pachyma cocos*)	3 grams
Bulb of *Arum pentaphyllum* boiled with the gall of an ox	6 grams
Peel of citron (*Citrus medica*)	4 grams

| Cinnabar (mercuric sulfide) | 10 grams |
| Root of wild yam (*Dioscorea villosa*) | 32 grams |

KIN-TING

Combine 1 gram of musk from the male musk deer (*Moschus moschiferous*) with 3 grams each of the following ingredients:

Ginseng root, peeled
Root of *p'ai chu* (*Atractylis ovata*)
Fou ling (*Pachyma cocos*)
Grilled root of wild yam (*Dioscorea villosa*)
Olibanum (frankincense)
Cinnabar (mercuric sulfide)
Brown ochre, macerated and then washed in warm water and dried seven times

Ginseng Leaves

Some Western sources maintain that ginseng leaves have no medicinal value; it is suggested that the leaves of such a Yang root may be super-Yin in nature. In China and Korea, however, the preserved leaves of the ginseng shrub, called *Shên-lu,* are sold separately from the root. Ginseng leaves may be dried in the open air, protected from direct sun, and stored in an airtight container. An infusion of Shên-lu is said to have emetic and expectorant properties.

Korean Medicaments

Korean medicine owes its origins to Chinese medicine, as shown by all retail pharmacy signs in Korea, which bear the inscription *sil-long-you-aup,* meaning "inherited medicine." Traditionally, both medical philosophies stress the importance of the gentle action of natural formulas.

The major use of ginseng (*In-sam* in Korean) is as an ingredient in tonics of various kinds. Sun Ju Lee, however, found a wide variety of peasant remedies in use in the Korean provinces, including ginseng-based remedies for acute gastritis, infant diarrhea, excessive thirst accompanying fever, chronic cough, anemia, alcoholism, abnormality of the blood, endometritis (inflammation of the lining of the uterus), nipple infection resulting from nursing, suppuration, furuncle (painful lump in the skin), toothache, malaria, hysteria, and general convalescence.

The following medicaments are taken from the Korean medical classic, *Pang-yak-hap-pyun.*

KOONG-RE-TANG'S GINSENG REMEDY

This preparation has long been held in esteem for treatment of dropsical conditions, in which excess fluid accumulates in the tissues. It contains:

> *Conioselinum univittatum* (a plant resembling angelica)
> Cardomom (*Elettaria cardamomum*)
> Mugwort (*Artemisia vulgaris*)
> *Atractylis ovata* (the Chinese *p'ai chu*)
> *Pinellia ternata* (the Chinese *pan-hsia*)
> Feverbush (*Lindera strychnifolia*)
> Licorice root (*Glycyrrhiza glabra*)
> Ginseng extract
> Cassia bark (*Cinnamomum cassia*)

KOREAN STOMACH MEDICINE

Prepared as a treatment for summer dyspepsia, this remedy acts as a stomachic to relieve indigestion.

Atractylis ovata (the Chinese *p'ai chu*)
Dried orange peel (*Citrus aurantium*)
Whiteleaf Japanese magnolia (*Magnolia hypoleuca*)
Pinellia ternata (the Chinese *pan-hsia*)
Cardamom (*Elettaria cardamomum*)
Ginseng powder
Licorice root (*Glycyrrhiza glabra*)
Betony (*Stachys betonica*)

E-CHUNG-TANG'S INTERNAL REMEDY

To control jaundice and vomiting:

Ginseng extract
Atractylis ovata (the Chinese *p'ai chu*)
Dried ginger (*Zingiber officinale*)
Licorice root (*Glycyrrhiza glabra*)

SAM-SO-UM'S COLD REMEDY

For colds accompanied by fever:

Ginseng extract
Perilla (*Perilla nankmensis*)
Angelica (*Angelica archangelica*)
Pinellia ternata (the Chinese *pan-hsia*)
Dried kudzubean (*Pueraria thunbegiana*)
Peel of bitter orange (*Citrus aurantium*)
Licorice root (*Glycyrrhiza glabra*)

Ginseng in India

Although true ginseng, *Panax ginseng*, does not grow in India, the folk medicine of this country has long included remedies based on two related plants, *Aralia pseudoginseng* and *Panax fruticosum*. According to an ancient medical classic of India, *A. pseudoginseng* acts as an aphrodisiac and stimulant; it is employed in medicaments for controlling vomiting and dyspepsia. *P. fruticosum,* which like true ginseng contains saponin, is used as a febrifuge (to reduce fever) and as an astringent.

Ginseng in Japan

Sakurazawa Nyoiti, known in the West as Georges Ohsawa, was a gentle promoter of the macrobiotic regimen as the true pathway to health of mind and body. According to Ohsawa, ginseng is the most Yang of herbs and his herbal preparation called Mu Tea is the most Yang of beverages. Mu Tea combines ginseng and fifteen other medicinal plants—peony, root of angelica, sea thistle, carthanne, rush, ginger, hoelen, japonica, licorice, cinnamon, bitter orange rind, rehmannial radix, moutan cortex, carophyll flos, and persical semen.[10]

Mu Tea is among the few authentic Oriental herbal preparations available commercially in the United States, generally in health food stores or other macrobiotic channels. It is marketed in individual foil packets by at least one company. Ohsawa recommends that Mu Tea be included in a regimen for rebuilding health in bodies weakened by Western diet and way of life, both of which may cause the body to become very Yin. Mu Tea will help to restore the natural balance of Yin and Yang forces in the body (the "Unique Principle" of macrobiotics). In addition to its general value, Mu Tea in combination with a macrobiotic regimen is suggested by Ohsawa for relief of headaches, influenza, and menstrual irregularities.

The California herbalist Masaru Toguchi studied traditional Oriental medicine under his grandfather,

Seiya Kikuyama, a "barefoot doctor" of Japan. He studied herbology and other natural therapies at the Kawasaki Institute of Scientific Research in Tokyo. Toguchi has collaborated with a Western physician, Dr. Sam Klein, in writing *Oriental Herbal Wisdom*.[11] Toguchi discusses traditional means of diagnosis and documents a wealth of herbal formulas used in ancient and modern Oriental herbal medicine. Ginseng is a component of many of his formulas, including preparations for the treatment of constipation, abnormal thirst, heavy bleeding, and assorted stomach problems.

Ginseng in Russia

During the Soviet occupation of North Korea after World War II (from 1945 to 1948), the USSR experienced firsthand the enthusiasm the Koreans accorded to the honorable ginseng. Curious about the efficacy of ginseng as a tonic and rejuvenator, the Russians sent a great deal of wild ginseng home for intensive study. The findings of the Soviet scientists were sufficient to make ginseng a hot property in the USSR. Today ginseng tonics and extracts are sold without prescription in most Soviet pharmacies, and popular belief in its tonic properties grows daily.

Ginseng was a fabled herb in Russia long before modern technology made its mark on the world, however. *Panax ginseng* is indigenous to the Sikhote-Alin Mountains of Siberia, and Siberian folk doctors have long relied on this herb for its tonic properties. These shamans, who have passed their knowledge from parent to child through many generations, call wild ginseng "the root of life" and praise its curative powers.

George St. George speculates that the most notorious person to emerge from among the Siberian shaman class was none other than Gregor Rasputin, archvillain of the Russian court of Nicholas and Alexandra:

> It is generally believed that the infamous Rasputin's ability to stop the Czarevich's [Alexis] hemorrhages, caused by hemophilia, was based on his use of some *ginseng* preparations, rather than on the power of his prayers. This is quite possible since Rasputin came from Siberia and, while in St. Petersburg, had formed a close personal friendship with Dr. Badmayer, the celebrated practitioner of Oriental medicine. Of course, this cannot be proved and must always remain a fascinating speculation.[12]

The experimental evidence delineated in Chapter 6 amply demonstrates the medicinal and constructive properties of ginseng. Modern Soviet scientists believe that it increases physical and mental efficiency and protects the body from damage due to stress. Therefore, the USSR has taken steps to ensure a bountiful supply of cultivated ginseng to supplement the rapidly dwindling wild crop and reduce the retail price of ginseng, which is exorbitant in most countries. Research on methods of cultivating ginseng has been applied to advantage on government-owned ginseng plantations; the largest is a specialized state farm called *Zhenshen.*

Further research has convinced Soviet scientists that another plant, *Eleutherococcus senticosus,* has much the same medicinal and constructive properties as Asiatic ginseng. In some ways this "new" herb may prove to be even more potent than *Panax ginseng.* Because it grows abundantly in the USSR, a panacea may soon be available at prices the common man can more easily afford. *Eleutherococcus senticosus*, popularly called Siberian ginseng, is already available in the United States (see Chapter 8).

Ginseng in North America

In Western medicine ginseng once was considered useful as a mild stomachic tonic, a demulcent, and a stimulant "useful in loss of appetite and in digestive affections that arise from mental and nervous exhaustion."[13] However, during the 1960s ginseng disappeared from the official *U.S. Pharmacopoeia*, a reflection of the general cynicism with which modern medicine long has viewed herbal medicine. But there are healthy signs that the burgeoning U.S.-China friendship will spur Western medicine to reexamine its roots.

The *American Journal of Chinese Medicine*, edited by Dr. Frederick Kao of the Downstate Medical Center in Brooklyn, New York, published its first issue in March 1973. Dr. Kao assures me that future issues of this professional journal will contain in-depth articles on herbal medicines, including ginseng. Such a journal cannot help but increase modern medicine's awareness of the potential inherent in natural remedies and non-Western therapeutics.

3

Asiatic Ginseng and the Siberian Challenger

From personal experience and observation I am assured that Asiatic ginseng is an active, strongly heating medicine. . . . Western people appear to regard the virtues of ginseng claimed by Orientals rather contemptuously—as imaginary and based on superstition. But the evidences are that the mystic value attached itself to ginseng *after* its virtues had been practically ascertained.

So WROTE William Carles from Seoul, where he served as consul to Korea at the turn of the century.

During the 1700s and 1800s occasional reports about ginseng drifted into America from missionaries and consular officials serving in Asia. They observed that the Chinese and Koreans persistently believed true Asiatic ginseng to have stimulative, tonic, and restorative properties, and that ginseng had been held in high esteem for centuries. In 1900 the president of the Chinese Merchants' Company of Shanghai, then one of the largest trading companies in the Orient, discussed the reputation of the herb:

> The Chinese have used ginseng for several thousand years; they know its value as a medicine; they use it in religious rites and ceremonies, and its use is as firmly established as their religion. They have been taught its benefits for generations; they have been taught that it possesses supernatural powers, and it is even worshipped. ... Ginseng is used by every Chinaman, no matter how poor.[1]

The Chinese believe that man and nature are governed by the same laws, and that disease arises from imbalance of the cosmic forces of Yin and Yang. Concomitantly, nature's tendency to create harmony suggests that nature must provide a remedy for every ill. This principle has led the Chinese to experiment with an astonishing variety of indigenous animate and inanimate materials in their empirical search for cures. For centuries their medical expertise was impeded by superstitious dread of the human corpse. It is said that a curious emperor once sentenced forty murderers to death by public vivisection—all in the interests of science. Despite the anatomical knowledge gained by this and doubtless other surreptitious dissections, Chinese medicine before the twentieth century remained steeped in superstition and folk magic. Nevertheless, modern science has shown that many native remedies—ginseng among them—cure by more than faith alone (see Chapter 6).

Cries in the Night

Many fabulous stories told in Asia describe extraordinary wild "plantations" of ginseng found by the guidance of a dream, a star, a beckoning voice. Such an extensive find would bring great wealth as well as health to the discoverer, and Chinese people apparently dream of finding ginseng in the same way Westerners seek the pot of gold at the end of the rainbow.

The resemblance of ginseng root to the figure of a man is reflected in the name given to the plant in most languages: *jen-shen* or *shen-seng* in Chinese, *in sam* in Korean, *chosen ninjin* in Japanese, and so on. Ancient Oriental astrologers linked ginseng to the man-figure constellation of Orion and believed that the astral influences of Orion would determine the potency of ginseng in each person.

A legend from the sixth century A.D. describes a miraculous event:

During the reign of Wenti of the Sui dynasty, at Shantang in Shensi, at the back of a certain person's house was heard each night the imploring voice of a man. When search was made for the source of the sound, at the distance of about a *li* there was seen a remarkable ginseng plant. Upon digging into the earth to the depth of five feet, a root was secured having the shape of a man with four extremities perfect—and it was this root that had been calling out in the night with a man's voice.[2]

In like manner, Chinese and Koreans have recorded their respect for ginseng through the ages. Billions of people over thousands of generations of a civilization imbued with high intelligence have praised ginseng. But only recently have scientists of both West and East discarded their cynical attitudes toward ginseng and begun to evaluate the fabled root according to the exacting demands of the scientific method.

Wild Roots

Ginseng grows naturally on mountainous or hilly forest slopes in the Manchurian region of China, North Korea, and the Sikhote-Alin mountains of easternmost Siberia in the USSR. The climate in these areas is rather dry and cold. The plant has never been common, thriving only in small patches in deep woodlands where its very specific cultural demands are naturally provided. The little root with its canopy of five-fingered leaves flourishes only in woods earth, protected from wind, rain, and sun by the forest roof of leafy boughs. It is found among hardwoods rather than conifers, and often associates in the wild with basswood (*Tilia*) and royal paulownia (*Paulownia tomentosa*) trees, with which it is supposed to have a mutualistic sympathy.

In China ginseng seekers still scour the most promising areas of Manchuria, particularly along the Chiang-pai Shan mountain range in southern Kirin province. In the past the ginseng regions were considered imperial preserves "kept free of the profanation of the vulgar herd,"[3] and annual forays by soldiers and camp followers kept the royal medicine chests well supplied. Manchurian, or imperial, ginseng—the finest available at any time—was reserved for the use of the upper crust of Chinese society, and the emperor often rewarded his favorites with gifts of ginseng. The lower classes made do with lesser qualities of ginseng; indeed, so fervent and pervasive was the faith in ginseng that trade in all grades was—and is—extraordinarily brisk. Ginseng is one product that has never been a glut on the market.

In days past, the root of wild Korean ginseng was reputed frequently to exceed twelve inches in length. This *san-sam,* or mountain ginseng, possessed enormous power. According to the American consul at Seoul in 1902, a single dose would cause a patient to lose consciousness for a period of time and to undergo a few weeks of considerable discomfort as a result of skin eruptions, boils, and other afflictions. But soon thereafter "rejuvenation" commenced, whereupon the skin cleared and the body became healthy enough to resist disease for many years.

Questionable claims such as this one no doubt contributed to the disbelief of most Westerners who had early experience with wild ginseng. Nevertheless, none of these observers could deny the unchallengeable faith of millions of Orientals, proved by the willingness of even the most impoverished to forgo basic comforts to purchase the expensive root.

Cultivated Roots

Because the scant wild population of ginseng comes nowhere near meeting the demand for its roots in any one year, ginseng has long been cultivated in China and Korea, and also in Japan, where Manchurian ginseng was introduced in olden times. Most Oriental ginseng plantations are under government control and ginseng trade is usually a government monopoly.

In Manchuria, North Korea, and Japan, the cultivation procedures are quite similar, as ginseng thrives only when its natural habitat is faithfully reproduced in the ginseng plantation. Asked to grow under normal herb garden conditions, ginseng soon shrivels and dies. Ginseng under cultivation in the Orient is grown from seed and sometimes from root cuttings. It is protected from the sun's rays by a low covering that may be removed at night or by permanent roofing that allows ventilation at all times. The most successful plantations use woods earth hauled to the farm or construct the ginseng beds right in the heart of the forest. Some Korean farms have developed a combination of leaf mulch and pulverized granite (*whang-t'o*, "medicine earth") that brings good results. Fertilization is limited to mulches of rotted leaves and wood (often of *Quercus sinensis*, the chestnut oak). The meticulous attention to detail required of the ginseng grower is illustrated by a description of a late-nineteenth-century Korean ginseng farm (*sam-po*):

> Each farm is a rectangular compound, one part containing the buildings inclosed by walls, the rest by hedges. The buildings, though built as usual of mud, stones, earthenware, and untrimmed timbers, and thatched, are strikingly superior to the other houses of the Korean people. . . . In each compound are one or more tall little

watch towers, in which a regular lookout is held over the farm to prevent raids of thieves, who might make off with paying amounts in handfuls of ginseng.

Beyond the buildings and occupying the remaining space in the compound are parallel rows of low, dark mat sheds, with roofs sloping downward toward the south or southwest. ... The row (or shed) nearest the houses is the seed bed for all the plants grown on the farm. . . . In the Korean ninth month (September-October) the seeds are stuck quite thickly in the seed bed to a depth of three inches in little watering trenches about three inches apart. Once in each three days' interval during its whole life the plant is watered, and the bed carefully inspected to prevent crowding, decay, and the ravages of worms and insects. The mat shed is kept closely shut, for ginseng will only grow in the dark or a very weak light. ...

In the second month of the second year after planting (February) the root is regarded as formed and the general shape of the plant above ground attained. ... The shape is nearly that of the matured plant. ... In the following February (of the third year) the seed plants are transplanted to the adjoining beds. . . . In this second bed the plants remain one year, and are then transplanted to the third bed, and planted still farther apart in their respective rows. A year later they are again transplanted, this time to their final beds, where they remain two and a half or three years. Generally speaking, seven years are required from the time of planting until the plant is matured. After its life in the seed bed, exacting care in keeping out the light is not so necessary, and I noticed the swinging mat was removed entirely from the fronts of sheds of plants in the final beds.[4]

The following description of a ginseng farm in China illustrates another common cultural method:

Two methods of cultivating ginseng are followed by the Chinese, viz., growing from seed, and transplanting young plants found in the wild state. A spot is selected in the dark, damp woods, generally where the soil is rich and loamy. The seeds are gathered when they drop from the plant to the ground. After the soil is dug over, these seeds are sown broadcast, and covered with dead leaves partially decomposed. This plantation they call their nursery. In from fifteen to eighteen months the young shoots appear above the ground, and as soon as they are two or three inches high, they are removed to the permanent plantation, and in three years more the roots are ready for the market. Whenever a root is taken from the ground a young plant is set in its place, so that a plantation once formed is producing all the time.[5]

The typical ginseng farm employs—and houses—a large number of peasant workers to give constant care to the plants. In addition to the demands of the six or seven crops of different-aged plants that must simultaneously be cultivated and frequently transplanted, the workers must maintain round-the-clock vigilance against theft of the valuable crop:

The garden has to be watched day and night. A watch tower is erected and the hands take turn-about in occupying the sentry posts. Another man continually patrols the garden during the hours of darkness. With a view to scaring off spirits and to prevent himself from feeling lonely, he makes the night hideous with his cries.[6]

Every ginseng garden or plantation must be registered with the government in Korea and in China. Growers are obliged to sell each year's crop directly to the government, which sets prices and determines distribution of the roots. Though a perfectly shaped, perfectly cured root may bring *ten times the price of gold* in the retail market, it is doubtful whether the growers are the beneficiaries of such enormous profits.

In Japan, Asiatic ginseng (*chosen ninjin*) is grown in the cool, fertile regions of Honshu. Five- to seven-year white, branching roots are sold as medicine in a dried, fragrant state called *ninjin,* some of which is exported to China.

Curing the Root

Ginseng is never sold just as it is when pulled from the earth. First the roots must be preserved by a process that concentrates the vital essence of the root and renders it powerful. The processing may take as long as forty days and may be done on the plantation or in a government curing house, depending on the locale. In any case the processing involves three major steps—washing, steaming, and drying—each of which is meticulously carried out.

Washing of the roots is usually done on the plantation. Each root is thoroughly washed by hand and brushed gently with soft brushes, often made of human hair. The object is to remove all particles of clinging earth without bruising or scraping the skin of the root. Care is taken that no rootlets or fibrils are broken off, for the intact root commands the highest price within its grade.

After washing, the creamy white or yellowish root must be steamed to achieve the appearance demanded by the market. In Korea and Japan all ginseng goes directly from washtub to steam basket, but in China the best quality cultivated roots and all wild roots are specially treated before steaming to produce a yellow, firm but flexible, translucent root highly prized as "imperial ginseng." Most of the recent sources impart an aura of mystery to this process of clarification, saying that the process is traditionally held secret by the ginseng growers and pharmacists. However, several descriptions of the process are available from older observers. Henry Miller, U.S. consul at Niuchwang, China, gave this report in 1904:

An ordinary rice bowl is filled half full of clean sugar (white or brown, according to the color to be imparted to the roots) and boiling water is poured thereon. When cool, the mixture is of a treacly consistency and it is then used for coating the roots, being applied by means of a soft brush. When coated the roots are laid on a piece of clean cloth, spread on the top of a grating over a pot of boiling water, a wooden lid or cap being placed over all. The steam ascending through the cloth softens the roots, which absorb part of the sugar, the remainder finding its way through the cloth into the boiling water, where it ultimately sinks to the bottom of the pot and recrystallizes. This sugar, not unlike taffy, has acquired a slight flavor of ginseng, and is sold as "ginseng sugar." During the steaming of the ginseng roots the coating of sugar is frequently applied, until they are sufficiently sweetened. They are then removed from the steamer and spread on trays to dry in a not too powerful sun.[7]

This time-honored system is probably still in use in China today. (America's superforager Euell Gibbons used a similar method to cure two wild roots of *Panax quinquefolium*, with excellent results.[8])

In Korea the washed roots are packed into baskets, which then are lowered into a covered earthenware steamer that sits atop an iron boiler fueled with pine wood. The roots are steamed for a variable length of time, determined by "the burning of a torch made of the fiber and bark of the locust tree. For seven-year old roots, 4½ inches are burnt; for six-year old, 3½ inches, and for five-year old, 2¾ inches. [This observer] suggested it would be easier to time the steaming by a watch and was told that easier it might be, but certainly not as reliable."[9]

After steaming, the roots are allowed to cool on mats in the sun. Then they are carried into an airtight drying house heated by charcoal fires. There the roots lie on racks for several hours, exposed to the carbonic oxide fumes released from the burning charcoal. Upon removal from the drying house, the roots are reddish and hardened. Further drying in the sun for at least ten days completes the curing process, during which each root has lost about two-thirds of its weight.

The Marketplace

Roots that mature entirely in the wild are the most sought after, and those from China are supposed to be superior to the Korean wild root. Since the native homes of ginseng in China and in Korea are divided only by the imaginary line of political inclination, the supremacy of the Chinese wild root is perhaps no more than a chauvinistic claim of the more ancient of the two cultures. Trade in all qualities of ginseng is brisk between China and Korea, though little of the wild root ever leaves its country of origin because of the extraordinary demand for it at home. Cultivated roots make up the bulk of the supply, and that supply includes roots imported from North America and Japan.

Ginseng is usually classified for trade in four grades or qualities:

1. Wild ginseng from China, called *imperial* or *Manchurian ginseng,* is the yellowish, translucent root of superior quality that fetches extravagant prices. The older the root, the higher its price, for the Chinese are in general great respecters of age. Price varies also according to shape of the root, and those most closely resembling the human form command the highest price. Accordingly, it is to Manchurian ginseng that the Chinese refer in the proberb: "Eat ginseng and ruin yourself."

2. Korean wild root and Chinese and Korean cultivated root is called *red ginseng* or *white ginseng* depending on the color imparted by the curing process. Red ginseng is usually the more valuable, but people in some districts of China prefer the white roots. In Korea it once was thought that white ginseng should be used only by men, being too strong for women and children, but this view seems to have become outmoded. Ginseng of the second grade is expensive, but not nearly so exorbitant as first-grade roots.

3. American wild and cultivated ginseng, a product of the North American species of ginseng (*Panax quinquefolium*), has been imported by China and Korea for the past 250 years.

The roots are white and unclarified (not translucent) (see Chapter 4).

4. Japanese cultivated ginseng is imported into China and Korea, where it is bought by the peasant classes or used to adulterate better-quality ginseng products.

The monetary value of Manchurian ginseng is legendary but certainly based on fact. A missionary in eighteenth-century China noted:

The places where the ginseng grows are on every side separated from the province of Quan-tong ... by a barrier of wooden stakes which encompasses the whole province, and about which guards continually patrol to hinder the Chinese from going out and looking for this root. Yet howsoever vigilant, their greediness after gain incites the Chinese to lurk about privately in these deserts, sometimes to the number of two or three thousand, at the hazard of losing their liberty and all the fruit of their labors if they are taken either as they go out of or come into the province.[10]

Ginseng of the second quality is very highly respected for its medicinal properties. Miraculous healing properties are ascribed to Manchurian and Korean ginseng, and it is absolutely believed in by all the people, from the highest to the lowest. Korea exports its ginseng to China, Japan, the United States, Canada, and Europe. No doubt there is also a brisk market in ginseng smuggled over the Korean-Chinese border.

From 1628 to 1860 the greatest ginseng market in the world was the Moon-chang in northeastern Manchuria, established at the close of the Ming dynasty. Although 330 miles from the nearest Korean prefect,

the Moon-chang ("door of trade") was the only point
in Chinese territory open to Korean merchants. The
trade mostly involved silk from China and ginseng
from Korea. An interesting facet of the Moon-chang
stems from the fact that the Chinese viewed the ancient Korean civilization as a budding young country
in comparison with the venerable age of China. The
Koreans sought the respect of the Chinese in order to
increase sales of their ginseng preparations and other
medicaments. But the Chinese—and most Koreans—
depended on the recently revised Chinese classic of
medicine, the *Pen-ts'ao Kang Mu,* which did not reflect medical advances the Koreans had made on
their own. To rectify this situation, a cunning scholar
named Whang-do-soon compiled a Korean classic of
medicine, the *Pang-yak-hap-pyun,* which included the
very preparations the Koreans hoped to sell to the
Chinese. To authenticate the Korean medicaments in
the minds of the Chinese, Whang-do-soon included a
clever preface that invoked the name of Confucius,
whom the author claimed to represent, thereby dis-
pelling all doubts of the Chinese and ensuring a
ready market for Korean medicines.

Despite the closeness of the Moon-chang to the Siberian border, there is little history of ginseng trade
between China or Korea and Russia. Nevertheless,
native ginseng has long moved in local trade within
Russia:

> Gin-seng can hardly be said to be an article of
> commerce in any of the coastal settlements. It is
> chiefly cultivated in the interior, towards the up-
> per waters of the Usuri, and the Manzas of the
> sea-board set quite an extravagant value upon it.
> I remember having once been asked $160 for a
> handful of roots by a native. He kept it carefully

preserved in a rich, black clay, wrapped up in birch bark. It was much whiter and more transparent than Japanese gin-seng and quite smooth on the surface. Near Hanka Lake gin-seng can be bought for a very moderate price; and further north on the coast I have seen living plants sold for three dollars or four dollars apiece.[11]

American ginseng does not interfere with the sales of Asian ginseng in the Orient, for the Orientals are firmly convinced of the superiority of their own native species. American ginseng is, however, generally taken as a spring tonic in Korea and China. Its general acceptability is illustrated by a 1917 advertisement in *Chinese Students Monthly,* which encouraged young Chinese studying in the States to send home to their parents a "most suitable" gift of American ginseng. The United States annually exports 100,-000 to 200,000 pounds of wild and cultivated roots to the Orient. Some purveyors of ginseng in this country suspect that American ginseng exported to Korea comes back to us labeled as Korean ginseng. If so, it is of little consequence medicinally, for although Orientals do not greatly value the medicinal properties of *Panax quinquefolium,* scientific tests have established its close similarity to Asian ginseng.

Tricks of the Trade

Wily schemes to make a few extra yen are not uncommon in the ginseng business. Certain species of *Campanula* and *Adenophora* may be offered as ginseng by unscrupulous merchants, for these roots do resemble the true *Panax* product. But these false roots are harder and woodier than ginseng, and an expert can readily detect the difference. Less knowledgeable buyers may employ a test to determine the identity of the proffered root. In one such test used in China, two men walk briskly together while one of them chews a bit of the root. If after a distance of three or four miles the man chewing the root has not tired but the other man is out of breath, the root is assumed to be ginseng.

Various other frauds are practiced, including the insertion of metal into the root core to increase the weight of the root. Few experienced buyers are taken in by this ruse. Another ploy involves tying hairs or silken threads around the rootstalk during the curing process, in order to produce crevices that resemble the year marks of the natural root. The dishonest merchant hopes by this means to fool the unwary buyer about the actual age of the root.

The New Wave of Oriental Medicine

The Cultural Revolution initiated in 1960 by Mao Tse-tung extended into all social and economic areas of Chinese life. The philosophical impetus provided by this movement stimulated an upheaval in the practice of medicine. Previously, modern Chinese scientists had concentrated their efforts in the few urban areas of China, and the "barefoot doctors" exclusively served the rest of the country. The medical knowledge of modern science did not sift down to the folk healers; nor did the folk remedies pique the curiosity of the "ivory tower" scientists. The Cultural Revolution forced the traditional and modern ways to intermingle, and Mao hailed traditional medicine as "a great treasure house" capable of yielding secrets unknown to modern medicine. Trained physicians worked side by side with the barefoot doctors, teaching them principles of modern medicine and in turn learning the fundamentals of acupuncture and herbal medicine.

Chinese physicians—long insulated from the wellsprings of native wisdom—were astonished at the effectiveness of the folk medicines. A research program was soon begun to test the multitude of herbal remedies in general use, and the researchers found that many preparations were based not on superstition but on the demonstrable curative properties of the herbs.

Today the medical profession has expanded to serve all parts of China, urban and rural alike. The medical system recognizes the value of the barefoot doctors and incorporates them into its multilevel structure. The native doctors practice as they always have, but now they are backed up by hospitals, clinics, and thoroughly competent medical teams. The eradication of dread diseases formerly widespread in China—cholera, smallpox, and venereal disease among them—is generally attributed to the new cooperation of traditional and modern medicine.

Respect for Oriental herb medicine has grown in the West as China has opened her doors to cultural exchange. Members of the Canadian Medical Association, for example, toured Peking's Institute of Pharmacology in April 1973 and were impressed with the work being done there in herbal medicine. Dr. John Evans, president of the University of Toronto, called Chinese herbalism "one of the world's richest medical resources." He went on to prophesy: "With 4,000 years of human experimentation behind them there is every reason to think that they may be able to develop a whole range of synthetic medicines of enormous potential for medicine in general."[12]

The New Discovery in the USSR

The Soviet Academy began three decades ago to

study native Chinese therapeutic processes. The Soviets believed that Chinese therapeutic medicine held herbal secrets that possibly would offer cures to some of the more stubborn diseases that plague mankind.

Soviet research into the composition and efficacy of ginseng proved its value as a tonic and restorative agent beyond all doubt. The eminent pharmacologist Dr. I. I. Brekhman predicted as long ago as 1957 that ginseng someday would be prescribed routinely for all people past the age of forty. He also thought it likely that the vitamin and mineral supplements of the future would contain ginseng.

The research results and the scarcity of ginseng prompted Soviet scientists to experiment with plants related to ginseng, in hopes of finding an abundant source of a similar "miracle tonic." Several years of experimentation with plants of the family Araliaceae proved that just such a source does exist. *Eleutherococcus senticosus* (Siberian ginseng), a shrubby plant related to ginseng, yields a chemical complex that has an effect on the human body remarkably similar to that of ginseng. Not only does *Eleutherococcus* strengthen the body and protect against disease, but it also has no known deleterious side effects. In fact, many Soviet scientists believe that it exceeds the efficacy of Asiatic ginseng in all areas.

Eleutherococcus has never been included in the traditional folk remedies of any people, despite its wide distribution and abundance in many parts of China, Korea, and the USSR.

Eleutherococcus is an erect shrub commonly called "touch-me-not" (*netronnik*, in Russian) or "devil's shrub" (*chiertov kust*) because of the prickly, downward-pointing thorns that thickly cover the young stems. The plant stands from six to ten feet in height, sometimes taller, and favors dense thickets of underbrush or shrubbery. The light gray or pale brown branches may lack thorns when the plant is mature. The compound leaves are borne on long stems; the leaflets are arranged palmately—like fingers on a hand, as are the leaves of ginseng—and bear tiny serrations ("teeth") and prickles on their margins. Short young plants with only three or four leaves could be mistaken for ginseng, but the two species do not generally grow in the same areas.

Clusters of small yellowish (female) or violet (male or bisexual) flowers appear in July. By September the blossoms have developed into nodding bunches of glossy black berries.

The succulent "roots" of *Eleutherococcus* are actually a shallow, spreading network of rhizomes (underground stems). The outer covering of the rhizome is pinkish-white, overlying a brownish yellow cortex and a small white pith. The rhizomes are slender, cylindrical, and branching. The odor of the rhizome, or root, is strong but agreeable, and the taste has a not unpleasant burning-spicy quality.

Unlike Asiatic ginseng, the leaves of *Eleutherococcus* have the same pharmacological powers as the roots. For this reason, only the leaves may be gathered from some plants, leaving the roots to propagate new plants vegetatively. This harvesting procedure is desirable because *Eleutherococcus* propagates very slowly from seed, and with limited success.

Eleutherococcus has a wide range of geographical and ecological distribution and occurs abundantly within that range, unlike the aristocratic nature of its rare and elusive cousin. It ranges between 35 and 53 degrees north latitude in the USSR, China, Korea, and Japan, encompassing the middle regions of Amurskaya Oblast in the USSR, extending east to Sakhalin Island and all of Japan, and stretching south to the Shensi and Hopeh provinces of China and the whole of South Korea. *Eleutherococcus* climbs mountains to a height of 2,500 feet above sea level, but it flourishes best in coniferous and mixed broadleaf forests at lower altitudes. It may form extensive thickets or stand alone, depending on conditions locally.

In spite of the vast natural supply of *Eleutherococcus* in the USSR, Soviet scientists have brought it under domestication to ensure a stable storehouse of this valuable plant. The Institute of Biologically Active Substances in Vladivostok has developed efficient methods of propagation and cultivation, both vegetatively and from seed. The pharmacological industry processes huge amounts of *Eleutherococcus* each year. The resulting products are widely used in the USSR and are exported to many countries. In the United States *Eleutherococcus*, usually called Siberian ginseng, is available in extract form and in premixed fruit drinks containing a one-day dose.

The Institute of Biologically Active Substances continues its examination of the botanical family Araliaceae. Many of its other species have been used medicinally in the Near and Far East for centuries. Only time and experimentation will tell how many of these species will prove useful in modern medicine.

4

The Ginseng Boom in America

AT THE TURN of the eighteenth century the enlightened Manchu emperor K'ang-hsi (reign, 1661–1722) welcomed the establishment of a Jesuit outpost in China, not so much for the religion it brought as for the scholarship and skills of the missionaries. For many years the bilingual Jesuit missionaries were tolerated at the imperial court, and K'ang-hsi employed their talents well. The Jesuits assisted as interpreters in state business involving Europeans, prepared elaborate maps, established the Chinese calendar, and performed many other services for K'ang-hsi.

In 1711 the Jesuit Father Jartoux was dispatched by K'ang-hsi to map a distant portion of the country. On his journey Father Jartoux experienced firsthand the healing wisdom of the Chinese people; in particular he was impressed with ginseng. In 1713 a letter from Father Jartoux reached the Royal Society of London. The missionary described "a Tartarian plant, called ginseng, with an account of its virtues." He noted that the Tartars called the plant *orhota*, meaning "chief of plants," and suggested, "If it is to be found in any other country in the world, it may be particularly in Canada, where the forests and mountains ... very much resemble those here."[1]

Jartoux's communication created little stir until it came to the attention of a Canadian missionary among the Iroquois in 1717. This priest, Father Joseph Francis Lafitau, was fascinated by Jartoux's description of the Chinese plant and his prediction of a Canadian counterpart. In his "Memoire ... concernant la précieuse plante du Ginseng," Lafitau wrote of his discovery:

> It was by accident that I discovered ginseng (after reading) with pleasure a letter from Father Jartoux. In it I found an exact description of the ginseng plant. . . . After spending three months looking for the ginseng, by accident I found it. It was ripe, and the color of the fruit at-

tracted my attention. I pulled it up, and with joy took it to an Indian I had engaged to help me hunt for it. She recognized it at once as one of the plants the Indians used.

The Iroquois word for the plant, *garentoquen*, signified an image of the lower body of a man with his legs held apart.

Lafitau was not the first to report the discovery of ginseng in North America. In 1704 Michael Sarrasin, King's physician for Canada appointed by Louis XIV, discovered the little shrub in the forests near Quebec and sent samples of it to Paris for examination. Nevertheless, it was Lafitau and his knowledge gained from Jartoux that led to the popular knowledge of the herb and the subsequent ginseng boom in North America.

Gathering Gold

Oddly enough, the French and English settlers were not interested in the medicinal value of ginseng for their own use. Fantastic stories spread rapidly among them about the fabulous prices paid for wild ginseng root in the Orient. Consequently, greed overpowered any idle curiosity about ginseng's healthful properties, and interest grew in the possibilities of trade with China. In 1720 the first company was formed in Canada to gather and ship ginseng to China, through Paris. For several years thereafter ginseng was second only to fur as an item of trade. Reports suggest that every able-bodied man, woman, and child set about combing the woodland slopes for ginseng. The more enterprising among them hired large groups of Indians to collect the wild roots.

The Canadian boom was remarkably short-lived, for the collectors in their lust for gold ignored the most basic tenets of conservation. They collected in all seasons, never allowing any plants to go to seed, and they rarely discriminated between young and old roots—all went into the collector's bag. As a result the wild stocks of ginseng thinned rapidly. Peter Kalm, the Swedish botanist, traveled through Quebec in 1759 and noted that the ginseng trade was still alive. But he predicted that the overzealous enthusiasm of the collectors would soon exterminate ginseng in its natural habitat.[2]

Early ginseng trade was very profitable to the French traders, who bought it from collectors for less than fifty cents a pound. The Company of the Indies resold it in China for as much as ten dollars a pound and so returned profits of ten- to twentyfold to the traders. But in 1754 the Chinese inspected several shipments of Canadian ginseng and found that the roots had been improperly dried and cured in haste and that a goodly proportion of the roots were not even ginseng. The reputation of Canadian ginseng was thus fouled by avarice, and the Chinese trade dwindled rapidly.

Colonial Roots in America

About 1750, when Canadian supplies of wild root were becoming scarce, trappers and traders spread the news of ginseng trade to the American colonies. Ginseng grew naturally throughout the forest areas of most colonial states, and the colonists were glad to have a source of extra income. At that time the easternmost communities of colonial America were rapidly maturing culturally, politically, and economically, but the farmers who moved north in New England or west to settle in the Allegheny range were still concerned mainly with survival. A day's foraging for ginseng could pay for seed for the spring crops or buy a new plow. Later, immigrants from England, Germany, Norway, and Sweden pushed past the Appalachian barrier and moved west to the Mississippi and north into Minnesota, encouraged by the land speculators of the 1800s. Many of the new farms were financed by heavy borrowing, and when drought and depression hit simultaneously in 1856, more than a few settlers survived by hunting ginseng.

A. R. Harding, buyer of furs and medicinal herbs, described the practice of the "sang diggers" who supplied the China trade:

> The sang diggers go into the woods with a small mattock, a sack and a lunch and the hunt for the valuable plant begins. Ginseng usually grows in patches. This is not because the plant is by nature a bedding plant but for the reason that the seeds fall near the parent plant. . . . In the early days, hunters found very large patches where for hundreds of years the parent plant and its progeny had increased without molestation. Sometimes as high as one hundred pounds of root would be secured from one such plot. Women as well as men and boys hunt the root. The plant is well known to all mountain lads and lasses and few are the mountain cabins that have no ginseng in them waiting for market.[3]

Adventurous men of vagabond spirit also supplied the ginseng market. They were the trappers, who kept one step ahead of the settlers in the push West and lived off the land and the profits to be made from selling furs and medicinal herbs. Itinerant buyers traveled through the wild frontier country, moving from Indian village to trapper shack to immigrant farmhouse, buying whatever furs and roots the people had collected. When a buyer had amassed a stockpile of such goods, he loaded his wares on horseback and began the arduous trek east. Manasseh Cutler in 1815 met one such traveler in Ohio "with ten packhorses, loaded principally with ginseng in barrels."[4]

As early as 1798 the French botanist André Michaux noted that ginseng was in jeopardy in many parts of its range as a result of the pressures of overcollecting.[5] Because the distribution of ginseng in the United States is considerably more extensive than in Canada, the natural supply was not as quickly exhausted, and wild roots continued to flow into the port cities throughout the nineteenth century. Indeed, the greatest year for the ginseng trade was 1862, when a total of 622,761 pounds of dried roots was shipped to Canton and Hong Kong. Nevertheless, by 1877 a few speculators began to think in terms of cultivating ginseng as a crop to augment the dwindling wild stock.

American traders paid twenty-five to forty cents a pound, and barrels of ginseng made their way on horseback over woodland trails to the eastern ports. The American export of ginseng to China appears to have taken up where Canada left off. In 1733 the sloop *Hingham* sailed from Boston to China with fifty-five tons of ginseng aboard. The *Empress of China* carried a hold full of ginseng to Canton in 1784, sailing via South Africa and the Canary Islands.

Captains of East India ships were impressed with stories of the aphrodisiac and tonic properties of ginseng. One of them remarked, "Those fat, luxurious mandarins are as fond as Solomon of wives and concubines, and are always adding a pretty little 'Peach Blossom' to their carnal collection. They *needed* the invigorating, rejuvenating herb ginseng."[6]

Natural Distribution

Before the ginseng boom decimated its stocks, *Panax quinquefolium* grew abundantly wherever conditions were favorable; its range encompassed every state from the Atlantic seaboard west to the states just across the Mississippi River, except for Florida and Louisiana. Ginseng was especially prolific in and around the Allegheny Mountains of Pennsylvania, Maryland, West Virginia, and Virginia. Though it followed the Appalachian chain to its southern limit, the plant was less abundant in the Carolinas, Alabama, and Georgia.

In appearance the plant closely mimics its Oriental cousin, growing under the cool protection of hardwood forests. Just like *Panax ginseng,* American ginseng takes at least seven years to mature its succulent man-shaped root, and the appearance of its leafy parts changes from year to year (see Chapter 7). After 1890 the legislatures of Virginia, West Virginia, New York, Ohio, Pennsylvania, Illinois, and Ontario, Canada, enacted laws for the protection of this endangered species. They variously defined the time of year for digging ginseng to prohibit taking the plant in spring and summer while it was producing its seeds. In this way the states sought to force the sang diggers to husband the supply of ginseng.

Colonial Medicine

Not all the ginseng yielded by the dense frontier forests found its way to the Orient. Many Indian tribes used ginseng medicinally (see Chapter 5), and their remedies often were adopted by white settlers. Because few physicians accompanied the Europeans who challenged the frontier, the settlers had to rely on half-remembered formulas and unfamiliar

American plants for their medicines. For this reason, "the Indian doctor, not altogether a charlatan or fakir, could always get a following, and any quack might be certain to receive, at worst, a tolerant hearing."[7]

Another source of medical care was the "yarb and root doctor," who traveled the frontier dispensing patent medicines based on native roots, barks, and herbs. These self-described "healers" had no formal training; most qualified as outright quacks, though a few felt they were answering the call and had the interests of their fellowman at heart. The people were at the mercy of these men, who preyed on their fears and took advantage of the lack of laws in the emergent communities. Virgil Vogel observes:

> Many of the early botanic physicians professed to have absorbed their knowledge directly from contact with the Indians. Some of them had indeed, by reason of captivity, trade, or other occasion for proximity with the natives, found opportunities to learn the red man's procedure and remedies. Some claimed to be at least partly of Indian descent. It was through these men that some of the Indian medical remedies passed to the whites.[8]

A combination of frontier wisdom and Indian lore is preserved in *The American Indian Doctor: Dr. John Williams' Last Legacy, A Useful Family Herbal.* The book, which appeared in 1827, offered several remedies containing ginseng. Dr. Williams found ginseng root to be an excellent medicine to ease "inward hurts and ulcers" when combined with equal parts of elecampane, comfrey, spikenard, angelica, and camomile, and two parts fir boughs, all steeped together in rum and water. As an "infallible remedy for wind colic in women and children," he recommended ginseng combined with white root (*Asclepias tuberosa*) and calamus or angelica—"very rare it ever fails."

The communities of the eastern colonies more often were blessed by the presence of a practicing physician. However, these European-trained doctors worked at a disadvantage when their imported medicines were unavailable. They were forced to act as their own pharmacists, experimenting and compounding medicines from the unfamiliar native flora. Indian lore seeped into even the most sophisticated physician's medicine bag as he sought information about the plants of this new country. One such physician, Dr. Fortescue Cuming, diagnosed malaria when asked to treat a young man of Marietta, Ohio. Cuming prescribed his own combination of a European herb, calomel, with native American snakeroot and ginseng.[9]

Medical care from any source in the colonies thus was unreliable. Many preferred to do their own doctoring, agreeing with William Byrd that priests, lawyers, and physicians were the three great scourges of mankind. Byrd, a Virginia planter and satirist, strode vigorously through a life that began in England in 1674 and ended seventy years later on his plantation near Richmond, which he founded. Scorning colonial doctors, he adopted nature as his physician. Ginseng was among his pet medications:

Though Practice will soon make a man of tolerable Vigour an able Footman, yet, as a Help to bear Fatigue I us'd to chew a Root of Ginseng as I Walk't along. This kept up my Spirits, and made me trip away as nimbly in my Jack-Boots as younger men cou'd in their Shoes. This Plant is in high Esteem in China, where it sells for its weight in Silver. Indeed it does not grow there, but in the Mountains of Tartary, to which place the emperor of China Sends 10,000 Men every Year on purpose to gather it. But it grows so scattering there, that even so many hands can bring home no great Quantity. . . . It grows also on the northern continent of America, near the Mountains, but as sparingly as Truth & Public Spirit. It answers exactly both to the Figure and vertues of that which grows in Tartary, so that there can be no doubt of its being the Same.

Its vertues are, that it gives an uncommon Warmth and Vigour to the Blood, and frisks the Spirit, beyond any other cordial. It chears the Heart even of a Man that has a bad Wife, and makes him look down with great Composure on the crosses of the World. It promotes insensible perspiration, dissolves all Phlegmatik and Viscous Humours, that are apt to obstruct the Narrow channels of the Nerves. It helps the Memory, and would quicken even Helvetian dulness. 'Tis friendly to the Lungs, much more than Scolding itself. It comforts the Stomach, and Strengthens the Bowels, preventing all Colicks and Fluxes. In one Word, it will make a Man live a great while, and very well while he does live. And what is more, it will even make Old Age amiable, by rendering it lively, chearful, and good-humour'd. However 'tis of little use in the Feats of Love, as a great prince once found, who hearing of its invigorating quality, sent as far as China for some of it, though his ladys could not boast of any Advantage thereby.[10]

Despite the high regard many colonists had for ginseng, its popularity waned and Americans began to feel that the Chinese claims for its potency were unwarranted. Whether this opinion arose because ginseng was touted for diseases it could not cure or because roots offered for use were underage, improperly cured, or not even ginseng, we can only speculate. Vogel reports the opinions of several who doubted the value of ginseng:

> Dr. Cullen ... called ginseng nothing more than a very mild aromatic and denied that it had the aphrodisiac powers claimed for it by the Chinese. Also cautious was the view of Jacob Bigelow, who held that the virtues of ginseng "do not appear, by any means, to justify the high estimation of it by the Chinese." ... By 1852 Dr. Clapp reported that ginseng was "seldom employed in this country."[11]

Ginseng remained on the official U.S. list of pharmaceuticals from 1842 to 1882 as a secondary drug for stomachic and stimulant uses. During the first half of the twentieth century, ginseng was officially listed as a demulcent. *Drug Topics Red Book* no longer lists ginseng at all, and it appears that whatever official uses ginseng once had in the United States are now filled by synthetic drugs. The pharmaceutical establishment in the United States has long down-rated the value of ginseng and other herb remedies, reasoning that their action is too mild to prove effective. Armed with medicinal bombs in the form of synthetic wonder drugs, they have lost respect for gentler, natural formulas that act over a period of time. But the Chinese believe, and Soviet experimentation is proving, that small daily doses of mild, natural tonics fortify the body and often perform "miracles" where harsher measures only aggravate.

Gardens of Prosperity

Human ingenuity rises to any challenge when money is to be made, and after the Civil War a few energetic men began to dream of fortunes to be built by supplying the Oriental ginseng market with home-grown roots. Wild ginseng was scarce at that time, and cultivated roots would be welcomed by dealers. Many sang hunters had tried to grow ginseng from seed or roots; all had failed. An old Cumberland Mountain sang digger commented on the situation in 1884:

> Sang's powerful sca'ce in these parts. People in Cincinnaty, Philadelfy, and more big towns has been a-sendin' of letters here for four or five summers, sayin' they'd give $3.00 first, then $4.00, then $5.00, and this summer they got her up to above $6.00 per pound, and they didn't get no powerful sight o' Sang nuther. . . . What's you goin' to do with Sang—plant hit? Mister, you's jist a-foolin' away your time. Sang won't grow 'cept in the woods. Hit's wild as a rattlesnake and won't be tamed. When you dig hit up once, that settles hit; mought jist as well dry hit, and ship hit to Chiney. Bein's hits all gone in the woods and is too wild to grow, we've done give up the Sang business.[12]

Undaunted by such warnings, one Wisconsin optimist set about raising ginseng from seed in 1877. After expending muscle and money and tender care, his crop failed totally—most of his seeds never even germinated. The following year the Botanical Gardens in Jamaica, West Indies, began an experimental cultivation program. Roots packed in soil and shipped from

Boston were replanted in the forests of Jamaica's mountains, but this project too soon failed.

The man who made cultivation of ginseng possible was George Stanton, a New York tinsmith whose motto was "Wear Out, Don't Rust Out." Too old to continue his trade in 1880, he began to look for a gentler source of the income and pleasure he had gained as a tinsmith. He learned that the amount of ginseng exports to China had fallen off considerably since 550,624 pounds were shipped out in 1876, and that the demand in China apparently was insatiable. Stanton had found his gentle trade.

George Stanton's Chinese Ginseng Farm was established in 1886. After reviewing the failures of other prospective growers, Stanton decided that ginseng could never be domesticated. Therefore he duplicated as best he could the wild conditions of ginseng's natural habitat. He hauled in woodland soil for his ginseng beds and built in provisions for shade that approximated the effects of the natural forest cover. He kept the beds ventilated and well drained and resisted fertilizing the plants with anything other than a mulch of forest leaves. To the astonishment of everyone but Stanton, his little plantation prospered.

Newspapers reported Stanton's success in glowing terms that engendered a rush of interest. A *New York Tribune* article in 1895 breathlessly reported, "You can make a fortune on a few square rods of shaded earth." Even among people far removed from such earthy concern, ginseng became something of a fad. The *Westminster Gazette* gossiped in 1894, "Amelie Rives is introducing Virginia ginseng diggers to politely-scandalised New York society."

Predictably, interest in cultivating ginseng for fabulous profits mounted rapidly, fed by advertisements of merchants eager to stimulate a new source of roots.

Their come-ons were at best irresponsible, for they described enormous profits to the grower without warning about the heavy labor required for success. Hundreds of people sent money to the merchants, who supplied them with seed and a promise to buy the resulting crop. Little ginseng farms sprang up like mushrooms after a rain. Enthusiasm waned as the farmers found that they must wait seven years before harvesting a crop. And even after years of devoted care, the crop could fall victim to one of many diseases.

Many discouraged farmers soon allowed their ginseng gardens to go to weed, but the more industrious cosseted their crops and waited for the roots to mature. Those who persevered made at least a small profit on their first harvest and stayed in business for several years. They were aided by research efforts of several state agricultural bureaus, notably those of Pennsylvania and Michigan in the early twentieth century. Banding together in national and state associations, the ginseng growers exchanged information and seed and lent one another moral support. By 1912 an estimated 150 acres were under ginseng cultivation.

George Stanton, father of the ginseng industry, presided over the New York State Ginseng Association for several years. He and others sponsored the *Ginseng Journal,* which merged with the *Goldenseal Bulletin* before 1900. The journal *Special Crops* absorbed both earlier publications in 1903 and appeared sporadically until 1935. It was devoted to information about cultivation and marketing of ginseng, goldenseal, and certain other medicinal plants, and served as a medium for exchange between growers.

The advertisements of ginseng merchants in *Special Crops* reflected fluctuating prices but a steady

Chinese demand. In 1922 an agent of William Boehner & Co., a New York firm still in business to-day, paid the Fromm brothers of Wisconsin more than $100,000 for their ginseng crop! The International Ginseng Company and David Blaustein of New York, Samuel Wells of Cincinnati, Becker Brothers of Chicago, and others vied for the crops of the ginseng growers. Most represented themselves as *the* principal dealer with strong connections in the Orient. David Blaustein's ad in an issue of *Special Crops* identified that company as "the largest dealers in the U.S. in ginseng, roots and barks." (The ad continues: "We deal too in beeswax, feathers, and old rubber boots and shoes.") The New York firm H.A. Schonen boasted, "We are the exclusive buying agents for the Shanghai Ginseng Syndicate, the most powerful dealers in existence in China." What the dealers did not advertise was the number of crops they refused to buy because the roots were undersized, diseased, or improperly cured.

The Depression turned most of the ginseng farms to dust. The farms that outlived the Depression died soon after their owners passed on, for it was the rare son who chose to follow his father's careworn path. Those few plantations that have been kept up and the new ones that emerge now and then continue to supply an average of 150,000 pounds of cultivated roots annually to the Oriental market.

The heart seems to have gone out of the ginseng business afer 1935. The association memberships dwindled and *Special Crops* ceased publication. Now interest is reviving, stimulated perhaps by the new American demand for Korean ginseng, which increases monthly. But boom times are special, and the aura of excitement that attended the first wave of interest in 1900 probably has died forever.

5

Drums Along the Seng Trail

PRIMITIVE MAN instinctively sought succor from the earth, and he relied on the plant world not only for food but for healing agents as well. Just as a deer may rub its wounded flank against the antiseptic sap of a sweet-gum tree, cave-dwelling early man gradually learned to use the various local herbs to ease life's little discomforts. What ills he could not relieve with plant drugs he "treated" with supplications to the spirit world and remedies containing two parts superstition for every part vegetable, animal, or mineral. Thus healing became intertwined with mysticism and magic, and in many cultures—Russian, Chinese, American Indian, and others—healing gradually became the province of the shamans, or medicine men, whose powers were attributed to the influence of various guardian spirits.

Characteristic of North American aboriginal religion in particular is its close association with the world of nature. The American tribes base most of their cultural patterns on the principle of unity with nature, and it is not surprising to learn that the various tribes turned their intimate knowledge of the plant world into an extensive body of medicinal lore. The plains and the forests served as medicine chest to the aborigines, who were careful to collect nature's healing gifts conservatively, gathering only what was needed and often replanting when they could. As in most primitive cultures, some medicinal plants were chosen according to the "doctrine of signatures"; for example, women of the Hopi tribe of Arizona drank an infusion of milkweed leaves to initiate the flow of milk from their breasts after childbirth. In America, as in the East, ginseng was one of the plants thought to be marked with a "sign"—the manlike shape of its root. But contrary to the Asians, who often combine several ingredients in their medicaments, most North American Indian plant remedies are based on a single herb.[1]

Wherever it grows, ginseng has been adopted by the native peoples as an aid in their battle against disease. In North America *Panax quinquefolium* appears in the herbal grab bag of almost every Indian tribe indigenous to the "ginseng belt," which extends from Maine to Minnesota and southward through the mountain chains toward Georgia and the Carolina coast. Many of these tribes are classified by ethnologists as part of the Algonkian language group, but their customs and folklore differ from tribe to tribe and their usage of ginseng must therefore be discussed separately. Though shreds of these once flourishing tribes still exist, their traditions regarding ginseng have been stifled by the restrictive and debilitating nature of reservation life—as indeed ginseng itself has been almost eradicated by the treadmill of industrialization.

The Ojibwa

The Ojibwa, or Chippewa, were a group of hunter-gatherers who originally dwelled in what is now Minnesota, Wisconsin, Michigan, North Dakota, Montana, and corresponding areas across the border in southern Canada. This is the Indian people romanticized by Longfellow in *The Song of Hiawatha*. Among the Ojibwa, as in several other Algonkian tribes, medical knowledge was held by a class of shamans called the Midewiwin, the "grand medicine society." The Midewiwin had an annual ceremony in which each member demonstrated his prowess. Each Mide, or priest, kept his own medicine bundle containing sacred objects—an ancient magician's bag of tricks believed to have powers of its own.

New members of the Midewiwin were selected only upon the death of an incumbent Mide. To become a Mide, the chosen candidate had to rise through several levels within the Midewiwin, during which time he consolidated his proficiency in the practice of medical magic under the tutelage of a Mide of great wisdom. According to W. J. Hoffman, the instruction embraced a résumé of the traditions of the Midewiwin, the various uses and properties of magic plants and compounds familiar to the teacher, and conversations relative to exploits performed in medication, incantation, and exorcism.[2] Thus the training is not unlike Carlos Castaneda's introduction into the world of a Yaqui medicine man, described in *The Teachings of Don Juan.*

An Ojibwa legend recounts the traditional version of that tribe's discovery of ginseng, which the Ojibwa employ against various ills. Hoffman offers this translation:

Once the daughter and grandson of an old Mide started out on a hunting trip, and, as the autumn was changing into winter, they erected a substantial wigwam. The snow began to fall and the cold increased, so they decided to remain and eat of their stores, game having been abundant and a good supply having been procured.

The son died; whereupon his mother immediately set out for the village to obtain help to restore him to life, as she believed her father, the chief priest of the Midewiwin, able to accomplish this.

When the woman informed her father of the death of her son, her brother, who was present, immediately set out in advance to render assistance. The chief priest then summoned three assistant Mide, and they accompanied his daughter to the place where the body of his dead grandson lay upon the floor of the wigiwam, covered with robes.

The chief Mide placed himself at the left shoulder of the dead boy, the next in rank at the right, while the two other assistants stationed themselves at the feet. Then the youngest Mide—he at the right foot of the deceased—began to chant a Mide song, which he repeated a second, a third, and a fourth time.

When he had finished, the Mide at the left foot sang a Mide song four times; then the Mide at the right shoulder of the body did the same, after which the chief Mide priest sang his song four times, whereupon there was a perceptible movement under the blanket, and as the limbs began to move the blanket was taken off, when the boy sat up. Being unable to speak, he made signs that he desired water, which was given to him.

The four Mide priests then chanted medicine songs, each preparing charmed remedies which were given to the boy to complete his recovery. The youngest Mide, standing at the foot of the patient, gave him four pinches of powder, which he was made to swallow; the Mide at the left foot did the same; then the Mide at the right shoulder did likewise, and he, in turn, was followed by the chief priest standing at the left shoulder of the boy; whereupon the convalescent immediately recovered his speech and said that during the time that his body had been in a trance his spirit had been in the "spirit land," and had learned of the "grand medicine."

The boy then narrated what his spirit had experienced during the trance, as follows: "He, the chief spirit of the Mide Society, gave us the grand medicine, and he has taught us how to use it. I have come back from the spirit land. There will be twelve [chief priests], all of whom will take wives; when the last of these is no longer without a wife, then will I die. That is the time. The Mide spirit taught us to do right. He gave us life and told us how to prolong it. These things he taught us, and gave us roots for medicine. I give to you medicine; if your head is sick, this medicine put upon it, if your body is sick, you will take it in."[3]

The legend suggests that the Mide used ginseng to prolong life and to relieve pain. Two more specific uses are described by Hoffman:

1. Small quantities of the powdered root are swallowed to relieve stomachic pains.
2. A person complaining with acute pains in any specific part of the body is given that part of the root corresponding to the part affected; e.g., for pleurisy, the side of the root is cut out, and an infusion given to relieve such pains; if one has pains in the lower extremities, the bifurcations of the root are employed; should the pains be in the thorax, the upper part of the root—corresponding to the chest— is used in a similar manner.[4]

This second application is a remarkable demonstration of primitive belief in the doctrine of signatures—like cures like. Indeed, the Ojibwa name for ginseng is "man root"—*Shte-na-bi-o-dzhi-bik.*

Huron H. Smith, author of several ethnobotanical studies of Algonkian tribes in the 1920s and 1930s, unwittingly documented the decline of an Ojibwa tradition. The Ojibwa encountered by Smith in the forest and lake regions of northern Wisconsin in the 1930s had lost all traces of the ginseng tradition described by Hoffman fifty years earlier. Smith found no medicinal use of ginseng among the Ojibwa. At that time they gathered it only for sale to white traders, who sent the roots on to dealers in products for the Asian trade. The people had even allowed *jissens*, an attempt to pronounce the English *ginseng*, to replace their native word for the herb. Whether the Ojibwa surrendered their ginseng tradition to a lust for "wampum" or whether their tradition simply subsided as a result of the dispersal of the people in the face of white men's progress, we will never know.

Whatever the case, the Ojibwa had not lost respect for the benefits of ginseng—be they health or gold. Smith tells us that they gathered the ginseng root only when its berries were ripe but had not yet dropped; then they pulled the root and planted the fruiting top deep into the root hole to ensure another harvest six years hence.[5]

The Menomini

The Menomini were a peaceable and industrious Algonkian tribe first encountered by European settlers as a hunter-gatherer culture inhabiting the northwest shore of Lake Michigan. Their village economy was based on gathering wild rice, fishing, hunting, and a very limited agriculture. Foragers were always on the lookout for the elusive ginseng plant, which the Menomini called *matcetasa,* the "little Indian," an allusion to the shape of the root. Huron Smith received a specimen of ginseng from a Menomini named Joe Pekore. This Indian's wife, Sophie, was respected for her healing talents, and ginseng was among her most powerful medicines. In fact, to ensure her supply, she dug it up in the woods and transplanted it to a corner of her garden covered by latticework. Sophie and other Menomini believed ginseng to be a general tonic and a strengthener of mental powers.[6]

The Forest Potawatomi

The Forest Potawatomi were an Algonkian tribe of Wisconsin forest Indians distantly related to the Ojibwa and Ottawa of the eastern woodlands. Potawatomi traditions suffered much transformation as this peaceful people was displaced first by the Iroquois, who pushed them westward, and then by the U.S. cavalry, who broke the cohesion of the tribe. The history of this tribe is tragic enough to suggest that its only remaining roots may well be herbal.

The Forest Potawatomi word *gisens* obviously was adopted from the English, and probably supplanted the word *wenane,* which is still in use among the Prairie Potawatomi.

When Huron Smith located the impoverished Forest Potawatomi in 1933 on a Wisconsin reservation, they still pounded their *gisens* root in pottery bowls reserved for preparation of medicaments. A poultice of ginseng was used to cure earache, and a ginseng infusion was applied to soothe sore eyes. Smith reports that the Potawatomi added powdered ginseng to many herbal preparations to mask the repellent flavor of the other ingredients.[7] (The taste of ginseng is not powerful, nor is it particularly pleasant—I doubt

that masking flavor was the real purpose of the ginseng here).

The Fox

The Fox Indians, another Algonkian tribe, call
themselves the Mesquaki (Meskwaki), or "Red Earth
People." This Wisconsin tribe (now relocated in
Tama, Ohio) developed a characteristic woodland
culture based on summer gardens tended by the
women and winter hunting forays over considerable
territory.

The Fox called ginseng *wenani,* meaning "calf of
leg," in the usual anthropomorphic reference. The
ground root was considered a universal remedy for
both children and adults, and was specifically used to
treat menstrual difficulties, stomach trouble, and excessive discharges of various sorts. One remedy for
flux (discharge) combined

> Flowers of water target (*Brasenia schreberi,* from
>   a pond in Green Bay, Wisconsin)
> Root of bloodroot (*Sanguinaria canadensis*)
> Inner bark of chokecherry (*Prunus virginiana*)
> Root of ginseng (*Panax quinquefolium*)
> Root of maidenhair (*Adiantum pedatum,* five-fin-
>   ger fern)

In this recipe, as in others of the Algonkian tribes, the
ginseng serves mainly as a "seasoner" to increase the
potency of the other ingredients.[8]

By 1928, when Huron Smith visited their community, the Fox had long gathered ginseng root mainly
for the high prices paid by traders. But even then a
Mesquaki woman in search of a husband was advised
to depend on a traditional ginseng preparation highly
recommended for spouse-catching. The formula for
this gentle potion called for ground ginseng, mica, gel-

atin, and snake meat. Apparently the battle of the sexes is universal, as reflected in the Fox name for this recipe: *pinahigani i'kwawagi ahaiyowatci ahunapamiwatci*—"a bagging agent women use to get a husband."[9]

The Cherokee

The Cherokee, an extensive tribe of Iroquoian lineage, inhabited about two hundred settlements in eastern Tennessee and the Carolinas before a smallpox epidemic wiped out half the Cherokee nation in 1650. Ravaged by a disease of the European colonists, against which the aborigines had absolutely no immunity, the Cherokee struggled to regain their tribal strength and preserve their culture against adulteration by outsiders. Most of the Cherokee were forced to undergo a calamitous relocation to northeastern Oklahoma during the winter of 1838–1839; during the long trek at least 25 percent of the tribe perished from exposure and disease. A few hundred Cherokee who had escaped the notice of the U.S. military fled to the hills of western North Carolina and established a new settlement. It was there that James Mooney studied the Cherokee in the 1880s under the auspices of the American Bureau of Ethnology.

The medicinal knowledge of the Cherokee was embodied in sacred formulas that laid down the tradition surrounding the application of remedies. Ginseng was called *atali-kuli*, or "it climbs the mountains," an allusion to the herb's habitats. In incantations that accompany the medicinal formulas, ginseng was addressed as "great man" or "little man," invoking the ancient like-cures-like superstition of the doctrine of signatures.

A decoction of ginseng root was administered by Cherokee medicine men to banish headache, muscular cramps, and other discomforts, including "female troubles." These remedies probably had real therapeutic value, but superstition clearly underlies the practice of blowing a wad of chewed root against the external site of an internal pain.[10]

In the 1880s the Cherokee sold large quantities of dried ginseng root to traders, who paid them about fifty cents a pound—nearly equivalent to two days' wages! As ginseng was fairly abundant in those days, a sharp-eyed hunter could gather a few pounds of roots in an afternoon and handsomely supplement his family earnings.

The Creeks

Originally a Muskogean people of Georgia and Alabama who subsisted on a maize-bean-squash agriculture supplemented by hunting, the Creeks early became "civilized" by the cultural influence of nearby colonial settlements and the U.S. policy of absorption and expansion. In spite of their socioeconomic transformation, the Creeks held on to many of their traditions, including their ginseng tradition.

A warm infusion of ginseng root was used to alleviate shortness of breath, croup in children, frailness, and what the Creeks call the "millipede disease," which causes the patient to cough profusely and become hoarse. According to John R. Swanton, the following formula—possibly meaningless—was said over the medicine used to cure shortness of breath: *Noki saladi noki leslai salati noki lesfank salati kaka kaka.*

To cure tonsillitis, parings of ginseng root and summer grape tendrils were steeped in hot water; a cloth soaked in this hot liquid was bound about the throat of the patient.

When a person was sick with fever and could not sweat, he was given a concoction of new ginseng

boiled with ginger obtained from traders and mixed
with a little alcohol. This preparation caused profuse
sweating and helped break the fever.

Superstition surrounds ginseng in the Creek tradition. Chewed root was applied to a wound to stop its
bleeding, but first the wound was cleaned out with
the long wing feather of a buzzard. Swanton tells us,
"At that time no one must be near, especially no
woman, and above all no woman at the time of her
monthly period."[11] A menstruating woman apparently
boded more danger to the bleeding warrior than the
quill of a carrion eater and scavenger. Miraculously, a
Creek named Jackson Lewis boasted of using ginseng
to cure a woman who had been shot in the head.

Fear of ghosts prevailed among the Creeks, and
several dread diseases were thought to "arise" from
dead bodies. The vicinity of a graveyard was a peril-
ous place for a Creek. When passing a graveyard,
therefore, a Creek took certain precautions to ward
off evil spirits and disease: he bit off a piece of ginseng root, chewed it, and spit it out on each side al-
ternately until he had spit four times each way.[12] This
done, he felt free to pass by the graveyard, secure in
the sway of the herb's protection.

For supernatural help in healing, the Creeks sometimes appealed to a male deity they called Yahola.
For example, if a warrior was shot and appeared to
be near death, ginseng was cut up and steeped in
a cup of water while the medicine man sang a song
invoking the name of Yahola and appealing to his aid
in the great emergency. Then the wounded man
drank the ginseng broth to prolong his life.[13]

Other Indian Uses of Ginseng

The Onandagas and Oneidas, Iroquoian tribes of
New York State, called ginseng *da-kien-tookeh* and

ka-lan-dag-gough, respectively, both meaning "forked plant." Apparently both tribes valued ginseng only for the money it brought from the French and English traders. The Onandagas ensured a good harvest of ginseng by sprinkling a bit of tobacco over the first plant found during a hunt; that first plant was left in the ground in hopes that a prosperous search would follow.[14]

The Alabama Indians took ginseng juice from the roots to heal sores. The Houma drank an infusion of ginseng to control vomiting and ease the pains of rheumatism. The Penobscots held a doctrine-of-signatures opinion of ginseng: an infusion of the "man root" was supposed to increase fertility in women.

Virgil Vogel conjectures that some of the Indian applications of ginseng arose purely from the importance the Chinese attached to this root.[15] The French and English traders who employed Indians to search out ginseng in the mountains impressed the scouts with tales of its curative powers—*and* with the price they were willing to pay for the strange little roots. It is not hard to imagine the Indian, who had always relied on nature's remedies, withholding a bit of the booty for himself and his family. Surely this was not the case among tribes with established ginseng traditions, such as the Creeks and the Ojibwa. But tribes such as the Menomini and the Penobscots may well have adopted this snippet of medicinal lore from the traders—just as the early colonists had come to depend on Indian medicines to replace the comforting teas and poultices unavailable in their new homeland.

6

The Evidence

SOCIOECONOMIC PATTERNS in the twentieth century
have tended to concentrate humanity in teeming urban masses. Man is exposed to stimuli of quantity and
quality such as no Cro-Magnon hunter could have
imagined. The constant assault of visual and aural
stimuli, the tremendous number of daily person-to-per-
son contacts that most every man, woman, and child
experiences, the pollution of our environments, and
the adulteration of our food and drink—all create a
stress pressure that the human body—stalled in the
time warp of evolution—cannot adequately handle.
Each stress saps the body's resources slightly; the
cumulative effect of modern-day bombardment of
stresses can be disastrous. Thus scientists interested in
preventive medicine now search for subtances that
will help the body adapt to a broad spectrum of emotional and physical stresses.

Among the stresses imposed on our bodies are
drugs designed to act in specific ways. Penicillin, aspirin, cocaine, cortisone, barbiturates, and other kinds
of drugs serve in the fight against pain and disease—
but every one of them has certain side effects that
damage one part of the body while the drug acts
positively on another part. The search for substances
that increase general resistance therefore has been
concentrated on those that are *not* accompanied by
deleterious side effects. Scientists call these valuable
substances *adaptogens*.

Research on adaptogens currently centers in the

USSR, although the medical establishments of other countries are also active. I. I. Brekhman and I. V. Dardymov offer the following requirements for preparations classed as adaptogens:

1. An adaptogen should be innocuous and cause minimal disorders in the physiological functions of an organism.
2. The action of an adaptogen should be nonspecific; that is, it should increase resistance to the adverse influences of a wide range of factors of physical, chemical, and biological nature.
3. An adaptogen should possess normalizing action irrespective of the direction of the previous pathological changes.[1]

Few substances meet these stringent requirements. All adaptogens under study are of plant origin, thus bearing out the theory that natural medicines are better for the natural body than synthetic substances, which almost without exception cause damage as they cure. The official Soviet press agency, Tass, announced in April 1973 that Soviet scientists are compiling a four-volume encyclopedia of medicinal herbs. More than a thousand medicinal herbs grow in Siberia alone. The Institute of Biologically Active Substances of the Siberian Department of the Academy of Sciences of the USSR, located in Vladivostok, has tested more than 200 of these medicinal plants.

Of all the adaptogens under examination in the USSR, *Eleutherococcus senticosus* and *Panax ginseng* meet the requirements most exactly. *Eleutherococcus* is popularly called "Siberian ginseng," because it is related to Asiatic ginseng (*Panax ginseng*) botanically and medicinally and because it grows most abundantly in Siberia (see Chapter 3). Both herbs have been scientifically proved to possess remarkable curative properties, as this chapter will show. Almost no experimental data exist for American ginseng, *Panax quinquefolium;* it has a composition similar to that of *Panax ginseng,* however, and thus may be supposed to share at least some of the properties of the Asiatic species.

Consequences of Stress

The Canadian physiologist Hans Selye proposed in 1946 a theory of stress that has since been fully confirmed. The human body reacts to every stress—no matter what its source, physical or emotional—in exactly the same manner. Stress may arise from a multitude of sources, including physical injury, invasion of bacteria or viruses, excessive heat or cold, emotional strain, nervousness, overwork, lack of sleep, malnutrition, excessive noise, polluted air, and chemical food additives. Exposure to multiple stresses may bring on disease—and the drugs, surgery, and X rays used to treat the disease constitute new sources of stress, not to mention worry over medical bills, concern for children and responsibilities, and fear for one's own well-being. René Dubos observes:

> Primitive man possessed automatic physiological mechanisms to enhance his chances for survival in the face of such threats as a wild beast or a human stranger. These mechanisms rapidly mobilized in his body a number of hormonal and chemical reactions facilitating flight or fight, safety or victory. Today the so-called flight or fight response . . . still comes into play when modern man finds himself in apparently threatening social situations. Stressful situations at the office or at a cocktail party elicit body responses

similar to those occurring during a competitive sporting event or actual fight; these responses occur even though the need to expend physical energy rarely arises.... [Modern man] must meet the challanges of today with biological equipment largely anachronistic. Many forms of organic and mental disease originate from the responses that man's Paleolithic nature makes to the conditions of modern life.[2]

Whatever the source, the reaction to the stress is the same. That reaction involves three principle organs—(1) the hypothalamus, a portion of the brain; (2) the pituitary, an endocrine gland lying beneath the central portion of the brain; and (3) the adrenal glands, which are endocrine glands that lie one atop each kidney. The hypothalamus receives notice of the existence of a stress from higher parts of the brain that monitor the body. The hypothalamus responds by secreting into the bloodstream substances (neurohormones) that are transported to the pituitary. The function of the pituitary is to regulate all the other endocrine glands. The neurohormones from the hypothalamus stimulate the pituitary to send instructions to the adrenal glands by means of a chemical messenger, or hormone, called ACTH (adrenocorticotrophin). ACTH is released into the bloodstream and is carried to the adrenal glands. In response, the adrenal cortex (outer area of the gland) secretes hormones called corticosteroids, which mobilize the body's carbohydrate, protein, and fat metabolism systems.

The interaction of hypothalamic, pituitary, and adrenal cortex hormones occurs continually in the normal body to maintain the normal balance of metabolism. But stress heightens the levels of each hormone and thus increases their effects. The emergency reaction to stress produces these results:

- Proteins, at first drawn from the thymus and lymph glands, are broken down to form sugar necessary for immediate energy.
- The blood sugar soars and the remaining sugar is stored in the liver in the form of body starch, or glycogen, which can be instantly converted into sugar if needed.
- The blood pressure increases.
- Minerals are drawn from the bones.
- Fats are mobilized from storage deposits.
- An abnormal amount of salt is retained.

Many other changes also take place to prepare the body to meet the emergency. Adelle Davis explains the ravages of prolonged stress:

If stress is prolonged after the thymus and lymph glands, whose proteins are purposely destroyed, have shriveled, proteins from the blood plasma, liver, kidneys, and other parts of the body are used. Stomach ulcers may occur not only because of increased production of hydrochloric acid, but also because proteins are stolen from the stomach walls. In ulcerative colitis, the destruction of protein brought about by prolonged stress literally eats away the lining of the intestine. During a single day of severe stress, the urinary loss of nitrogen has shown that the amount of body protein destroyed equals that supplied by four quarts of milk.

In the same way that the body suffers when its proteins are necessarily stolen and not replaced, so are the bones weakened by the theft of calcium. Dozens of other destructive changes similarly occur. Increased blood pressure alone may become dangerous. It is extremely important, therefore, for each of us to learn how to protect ourselves from the ravages of stress.[3]

Very many sources of stress exist today that did not exist when the stress mechanism evolved. Consequently, our bodies are forced by their reactions to everyday phenomena to function at an almost continual emergency level. The results are seen all around us in the unprecedented numbers of people afflicted with nervous disorders, stomach ulcers, colitis, cancer —the list seems endless.

What Adaptogens Do

The value of adaptogens lies in their ability to increase nonspecific resistance to stress. Adaptogens stimulate the central and peripheral nervous systems and thus affect every part of the body, directly or indirectly. Both Siberian ginseng (*Eleutherococcus*) and *Panax ginseng* enable the body to bounce back: They contribute to a more sparing use of carbohydrates and a rebuilding of glycogen reserves and high-energy phosphorus compounds.[4] This rebuilding of nutrients, called *anabolism,* prepares the body for the next onslaught of stress. Brekhman and Dardymov cite evidence that patients taking ginseng show increased body weight after prolonged illness, rebuilding of blood components after massive bleeding, and strengthening of the immunity mechanism.[5]

Certain steroid drugs also can stimulate anabolism in the human body, but they do so whether or not stress exists and thus may overload the system; *and* they produce unfortunate side effects such as masculine body changes in women (coarsening of hair, deepening of voice, etc.). Siberian and Asiatic ginseng, on the other hand, act only in the presence of "an appropriate background"—that is, when they are needed—and they have no undesirable side effects.[6] Taken daily in small doses, these adaptogens are like a personal bodyguard, ever ready to rise to your defense, but hanging in the background until summoned.

Unlike synthetic drugs designed to act against a specific disease condition, Siberian and Asiatic ginseng work in a nonspecific manner and thus are valuable agents against a broad spectrum of clinical disorders. They set up a universal defense system capable of increasing the body's resistance to physical factors such as overheating and radiation, to chemical factors such as poisons and cancer-inducing substances, and to biological factors such as bacteria and viruses.[7]

Normalizing Effect of Adaptogens

In the normal body a system of metabolic mechanisms operates to maintain a considerable constancy of conditions within the body. That constancy is called *homeostasis*. Many conditions in the body are so constant that persistent minor departures from the normal indicate a disease condition. Thus in man the body temperature, the amount of sugar in the blood, the concentration of salts in bodily fluids, the number of red and white blood cells, and many other factors are constant or vary only within narrow limits. By and large it is the internal environment that is kept constant. The body cells are thus helped indirectly to have a constant composition and level of activity—or, at least, to return quickly to normal if temporarily altered. These mechanisms operate hand in hand with the body's phenomena of adaptation.

Both Siberian and Asiatic ginseng promote the return of the body to a normal, healthy condition—*no*

*matter what pathological changes are occurring in
the body* previous to the administration of the adaptogen. Experimental evidence proves that both species impede damage to the adrenals and to the thyroid gland and reduce sugar levels in hyperglycemia
(too much sugar in blood) *and* increase sugar levels
in hypoglycemia (too little sugar in blood).[8] The fact
that these adaptogens can beneficially affect two directly opposite conditions such as hyperglycemia and
hypoglycemia is convincing evidence of their truly remarkable normalizing homeostatic ability.

Normalizing action was also observed in cases of
both disease-caused increase and decrease of red and
white blood cells.[9] Other evidence of normalizing action of *Eleutherococcus* and *Panax ginseng* are discussed in specific contexts below.

How Do Adaptogens Work?

Soviet scientists were astonished at the range of
beneficial effects of Siberian and Asiatic ginseng that
showed up in their early studies with these adaptogens. Unable to account for such a broad spectrum of
action, they set out to determine how ginseng produces these effects.

It soon became clear that both ginseng preparations
*alter the body's anatomical and biochemical responses
characteristic of the alarm stage of stress*: specifically,
they reduce the activation of the adrenal cortex, limit
the shriveling of the thymus and lymph glands, reduce the number of bleeding ulcers in the stomach,
and lessen other destructive processes.[10]

For reasons not yet understood, this antialarm action does not diminish the body's resistance to stress.
Paradoxically, the antialarm action and the nonspecific increased resistance to stress occur simultaneously
after *Eleutherococcus* or *Panax ginseng* are taken.

The mechanism that allows this dual effect remains unexplained. But the results of the dual effect are undeniable: *Siberian and Asiatic ginseng enable the body to fight stress without suffering the degenerative effects that usually occur when the body's response to stress is prolonged.* For this reason these adaptogens are suited to regular use to ward off the effects of stress.

The universality of the action of *Eleutherococcus* and *Panax ginseng* is indicated by the results of experimental research outlined below.

Stimulation of Work Efficiency

Because mental and physical work brings into play almost all the physiological systems of the human body, a man's capacity for work is a very good indicator of his overall functional condition. According to Dr. Bruce Halstead, Soviet astronauts take Siberian or Asiatic ginseng to improve their endurance in space.[11] Siberian and Asiatic ginseng stimulate increased work ability and efficiency in experimental animals and in man.

A German medical journal reports that administration of ginseng extract increased the work capacity of swimming mice by 35 percent.[12] Russian studies show that *Eleutherococcus* increases work capacity in experimental animals by 25 to 70 percent, depending on the strength of the preparation given.[13]

Experiments with people suggest that Siberian and Asiatic ginseng increase both the quantity and the quality of work output. *Eleutherococcus* in particular improves fine coordination of movement as well as work efficiency. It increases perceptivity of the sense organs and has been definitely shown to improve acuity of sight and hearing.[14] These effects probably stem from overall stimulation of the central nervous system that follows use of Siberian or Asiatic ginseng.[15]

Brekhman describes the results of one series of tests on Siberian ginseng:

> To study the peculiarities of the *stimulating and toning* effect of Eleutherococcus on man's occupational activity, observations of the work of radiotelegraph operators were carried out. It is known that this work makes high and diverse demands of the organism, such as deep concentration of attention, quickness of reaction, exact coordination of movements, high acuity of audition and vision. Besides mental efforts the work of a radiotelegraph operator requires great physical endurance. Eleutherococcus has appeared not only to increase the working capacity of the operators, but also to reduce the number of mistakes. The improvement of the operators' performances was evidently due to the general and diverse effect of Eleutherococcus upon various functions of the organism, beginning from muscular and ending with cortical ones.
>
> Thus, Eleutherococcus quite satisfactorily meets the demands made of stimulants and toning remedies. The possibility of using it in conditions of man's everyday work is determined by its capacity to improve the quantitative and qualitative performances of man's work, to relieve signs of fatigue, to eliminate various vegetative shifts developing not only in comfort conditions but also under the action of various adverse environmental factors, as well as by the absence of excitatory effect and, at last, absolute safety.[16]

Among the general metabolic effects of *Panax ginseng* is a complex of phenomena that work to increase energy buildup in the body and to bring about a minimum expenditure of energy. In addition, ginseng apparently contributes to muscular efficiency in humans by as much as 40 percent. Adaptogens also enhance work capacity and reduce fatigue under arduous conditions such as severe temperatures and long hours. Remarkably, *Eleutherococcus* and *Panax ginseng* stimulate work efficiency *without* inducing the nervousness, excitability, or sleeplessness characteristic of synthetic drugs such as amphetamines. In fact, the stimulating action of Siberian and Asiatic ginseng most often is accompanied by increased appetite, weight gain, improved sleep habits, and increased levels of hemoglobin in the blood—all signs of a healthy, relaxed body. This gentle strength results from the normalizing effect of the adaptogens.

Protection Against Alcohol and Other Poisons

Panax ginseng and *Eleutherococcus* protect the body against poisonous effects of chemical compounds, including ether, chloral hydrate, aminazine, barbital, chlorpromazine, and urethane. P. P. Golikov found that mice injected with ginseng extracts were much better able to resist the killing effects of strychnine than were mice unprotected with ginseng.[17] Brekhman cites evidence that Asiatic and Siberian ginseng reduce the toxic effects of synthetic drugs, thus allowing them to act against specific disorders without harming the body. Such evidence suggests that Siberian and Asiatic ginseng may protect the body not only from the toxic effects of drugs but also from the ravages of the food additives and pollutants to which we are constantly exposed. N. V. Lazarev has had good results using *Eleutherococcus* to reduce the toxicity of an important antitumor drug.[18]

Alcohol, the greatest problem "drug" in the United

States, also is among the most dangerous because of its widespread destructive effects on body tissues. In the excessive drinker, the stomach and intestinal linings become inflamed, nausea occurs regularly, nerves in the extremities degenerate, and the liver undergoes severe changes. Lesser changes occur in the moderate drinker, of course, but alcohol works its poisonous effects even in small doses. Experimental data suggest that *Panax ginseng* and *Eleutherococcus* protect the body against the toxic effect of alcohol.[19] In addition, both traditional and modern opinions hold that ginseng encourages rapid recovery from hangover, perhaps because of its normalizing action.

Functional Nervous Disorders

Clinical observations show that *Panax ginseng* and *Eleutherococcus* bring relief to people suffering from nervous and psychic disturbances, including neuroses, hypochondriacal states, and nervous instability accompanying male climacteric and female menopause.

The normalizing action of the adaptogens eliminates or relieves depression and neurotic fatigue. Brekhman notes that a three- to four-week course of treatment with *Eleutherococcus*

> . . . produced a sedative effect upon emotionally excited patients, made their mood calm and balanced, stimulated their interest in life and work. . . . Objective findings and the patients' good self-feeling pointed to a pronounced therapeutic effect produced by *Eleutherococcus* in the treatment of functional nervous disorders. . . . The therapeutic effect of *Eleutherococcus* is rather stabilizing.[20]

Tranquilizing, sedative, and antidepression effects of

Panax ginseng also have been experimentally obtained by several researchers.[21]

Cardiovascular and Blood Disorders

The overall tonic action of *Panax ginseng* and *Eleutherococcus* has beneficial effects on various diseases involving the heart and blood vessels, including rheumatic heart disease, hypotension, atherosclerosis, and mild hypertension. A. P. Golikov carried out a series of tests on atherosclerotic patients in Leningrad. Atherosclerosis is a disease process in which the major blood vessels are gradually closed off by deposits of fat and minerals; patients complain of chest pains, weakness, and general fatigue. After one month of treatment with *Eleutherococcus* extract, the patients showed marked improvement; weakness and fatigue lessened and chest pains and headaches were relieved. Golikov reported, "The treatment with *Eleutherococcus* was accompanied by an improvement of coronary circulation, normalization of the arterial pressure, favorable shifts in protein and lipid [fat] metabolism, and a reduction of serum cholesterol."[22] *Panax ginseng* reduces absorption of cholesterol from the stomach and intestines and reduces bodily retention of cholesterol taken in (eaten) or produced by the body.[23] These actions contribute to prevention or improvement of atherosclerotic conditions, as does the increased coronary blood flow observed following administration of *Panax ginseng* in several species of animals.

Eleutherococcus and *Panax ginseng* exert their normalizing effect to raise blood pressure in hypotensive patients and reduce blood pressure in hypertensive patients. Neither adaptogen is recommended for use in cases of severe hypertension, however. Patients suffering from rheumatic and other cardiovascular diseases showed improved physical and mental condition after four weeks of ginseng therapy.

Panax ginseng has tonic effects on the composition of the blood. Increased concentrations of red blood cells and the materials involved in the manufacture of red blood cells (iron, hemoglobin, erythropoietin, and so on) have been noted in experimental animals dosed with ginseng.[24]

Diabetes

In laboratory tests with rats, diabetes (induced by injections of alloxan) caused loss of body weight and high concentrations of sugar in the urine. Treatment with either species of ginseng stopped weight loss, reduced the level of sugar in the urine, and doubled or tripled the average length of life of the rats.[25] Similar results with laboratory animals are cited by Tagaki, Saito, and Tsuchiya and by K. A. Meschcherskaya.[26]

In therapeutic tests on patients with diabetes of light to moderate severity, Brekhman found that *Eleutherococcus* caused reduction of the blood sugar level. Treatment was markedly successful in the case of one female patient: After four weeks of *Eleutherococcus* treatment, her blood sugar level was reduced by almost 40 percent and urine sugar gradually reduced from 4 percent to 0.5 percent. Most of Brekhman's patients showed considerable improvement in general health, felt stronger and tired less easily, and experienced relief from the thirst and itching characteristic of diabetes.

Other tests show that blood sugar decreases after oral administration of Asiatic ginseng (hypoglycemic effect) in normal laboratory animals and in those with abnormally high levels of blood sugar (diabetes). Ginseng also increased blood sugar levels to counteract hypoglycemia induced by administration of excess insulin.

Cancer

Recently Soviet and American investigators have conducted many experiments to determine the antitumor properties of *Panax ginseng* and *Eleutherococcus*. N. V. Lazarev reported in 1963 that ginseng extracts inhibit the growth of malignant tumors in mice by as much as 48 percent.[27] Since then, other tests have shown that *Eleutherococcus* inhibits tumors in connective tissue, lung tumors in mice,[28] thyroid gland tumors in rats, and the spreading of cancerous growths in other laboratory animals. The formation of spontaneous mammary gland tumors has been experimentally inhibited in mice. When tumors were transplanted into the bodies of mice previously injected with *Eleutherococcus*, the tumors were less likely to take hold, compared with tumors in mice unprotected by *Eleutherococcus*. *Panax ginseng* shows positive effects similar to those of *Eleutherococcus* but less potent.[29]

Cancer develops most frequently in persons with weakened resistance. In light of this fact and experimental results, scientists have concluded that the way to cancer control lies in general strengthening of bodily resistance in combination with direct drug therapy or radiation therapy at the site of malignant growth. An adaptogen such as *Eleutherococcus* or *Panax ginseng* appears to be perfectly suited for use in increasing resistance to cancer not only because of its normalizing and stress-resistant action but also because of its antitoxic effect against strong synthetic drugs and radiation poisoning.

In addition, research has shown the following positive effects of Siberian ginseng against tumorous conditions. *Eleutherococcus*

- Retards the growth of adenomas (usually benign tumors of the epithelium).
- Wards off tumors caused by hormonal or endocrine disturbances, by relieving the precancerous condition.
- Inhibits the development of new sites of tumorous growth (metastases).
- Improves the outlook for radiation therapy.
- Inhibits relapses after successful treatment with drugs or radiation.

Panax ginseng has shown similar antitumor effects in specific situations, such as inhibiting growth of adrenal tumors in mice.

Brekhman concludes from the results of experimental cancer research that Siberian ginseng

counteracts the processes of induction and transplantation of malignant tumors and metastatic dissemination of malignant tumors and potentiates the specific effect of antitumor agents. . . . *Eleutherococcus* is a potent and safe stimulant which is especially needed by (cancer) patients. Its antitoxic effect will enable the patients to endure better the treatment with anticancer medicines, which are far from being safe for the organism. Even in patients with the third-stage cancer, whose state was grave, an improvement of mood, general state, and appetite could be achieved with three or four doses of *Eleutherococcus*. The arterial pressure, pulse, and respiration rate in *Eleutherococcus*-treated patients were much better than in control patients observed in parallel. No side effects were noted in any case. The authors have come to a conclusion that it is expedient to carry out further studies of *Eleutherococcus* as an important constituent of the complex therapy of cancer.[30]

Radiation Poisoning

Radiation therapy and diagnostic X rays can have very harmful effects on the human body. Radiation poisoning produces bodily effects including genetic and structural damage to cells in the blood-forming tissues, the skin, the lining of the intestines, and the sperm-forming tissues. A well-established long-term effect of radiation exposure on laboratory animals is shortening of the life span (deleterious effects of radiation are the result of free radicals produced by irradiation, discussed below). Because of these adverse effects, most physicians are reluctant to use radiation therapy unless absolutely necessary. But diagnostic X rays are administered more freely, and it is a wise person who keeps track of the amount of X rays he receives. Everyone of us is constantly exposed to "background radiation" arising from natural sources. High-voltage power supplies for radar and television, seepage from underground nuclear tests, radioactive contamination of food and drinking water, microwave ovens, luminous-dial watches, and even phonographic static reducers may emit sufficient radiation to cause concern.

Research has proved that both Siberian and Asiatic ginseng significantly reduce the damaging effects of radiation. Radioprotective and medicinal action of these adaptogens is effective against short-term and long-term exposure to radiation. In prolonged irradiation, *Panax ginseng* and *Eleutherococcus* doubled the life expectancy of rats and improved blood composition.[31]

Brekhman noted the following results when Siberian ginseng was given prior to antitumor radiation therapy: "The use of *Eleutherococcus* for prophylactic purposes (against radiation sickness) makes the body more resistant to radiation and enables the physician to use higher doses of radiation without severe complications."[32]

Body-Building Tonic Action

Both species of ginseng contribute to general health and strength by helping to rebuild vital tissues. In experiments with farm animals given *Eleutherococcus*, body weight began to increase after two weeks. Blood donors who take ginseng daily after giving blood achieve normal blood hemoglobin levels two or three times faster than blood donors who do not take ginseng. Patients suffering from emaciation or chronic disorders experience general strengthening of body tone and weight gain after they are given Siberian ginseng.[33]

Asiatic ginseng stimulates rapid rebuilding of the blood following hemorrhage and has a beneficial effect on the formation of red blood cells in starving rats. In experiments on rabbits, liquid extracts of Asiatic or Siberian ginseng increased manufacture of nutrients in the body and therefore improved general body condition.[34]

Though experiments with humans have not yet been extensively made, the results of animal experimentation tend to substantiate what Eastern folk doctors have long maintained: Ginseng strengthens the bodies of sick people and keeps healthy people healthy. To judge from the experimental results, ginseng should be valuable medicine for convalescents, facilitating their rapid recovery. It is also useful in correcting nutritional disorders, for it increases the tone of the digestive tract and enhances protein, carbohydrate, and fat metabolism.

Cellular Metabolism

Asiatic and Siberian ginseng have beneficial effects on several metabolic processes at the cellular level. In addition, they prolong the life of cells removed from the body. Animal experiments have produced the following results. Ginseng has been found to

- Provoke the normal growth of skin cells in albino rats and their regeneration after radiation injury.
- Accelerate synthesis of DNA in skin cells.
- Stimulate RNA synthesis in liver cells.
- Expedite DNA synthesis in lymphocytes under normal and stressed conditions.
- Tend to increase DNA/RNA content of adrenal cells.
- Enhance formation of ATP (energy factor).[35]

These stimulants to cellular metabolism no doubt are the source of the adaptogenic effects of *Panax ginseng* and *Eleutherococcus* and ultimately of their contribution to longevity, as well as to regeneration and wound healing. Much research remains to be done on the precise cellular action of both species.

Brekhman notes that *Eleutherococcus* and *Panax ginseng* promote antiradical and antioxidant reactions in the body.[36] It is thought that free radicals produce disturbances in the body that lead to internal stress, cancer, aging, and other destructive processes. A radical is a group of atoms that enters into and goes out of chemical combination without change; it is one of the fundamental constituents of many molecules. Certain destructive forces such as irradiation may cause the breaking away of radicals from a molecule; these are called *free radicals*. Free radicals can also be formed by oxidation of a molecule—that is, an oxygen atom attaches to a molecule, displacing the radical and setting it free. Oxidation occurs readily in the normal body. Any resulting free radicals "wander" about in the body until they attach to another molecule, thus altering that molecule's normal composition. The altered molecule can no longer carry out its appointed task in the body chemistry. If that task is part of the mechanism of gene synthesis or enzyme synthesis, the body's workings can be seriously impaired, because it is the genes and the enzymes that direct all the bodily functions.

Many scientists suspect that the cumulative effect of free-radical damage is the cause of aging. The human body gradually and constantly renews itself by replacing its parts through cell duplication and proliferation. Thus there is no real reason for a healthy and well-cared-for body to deteriorate—*unless* the instructions for cell reproduction become muddled by mutation, the effects of free radicals, or other means. The fact that *Panax ginseng* and *Eleutherococcus* reduce oxidation and the formation of free radicals means that these adaptogens prevent some of the wear and tear of living and may well contribute to longevity.

Fertility and Fecundity

At least one group of researchers has obtained evidence that Asiatic ginseng may at least slightly increase fertility. The group administered extracts of *Panax ginseng* and hormones to patients complaining of sterility. Increase of sperm count occurred in 28.5 percent of the men, and successful impregnation of their partners followed in 10 percent of the cases.[37]

Numerous experiments with minks have shown that *Eleutherococcus* diminishes the number of sterile females and reduces by half the number of stillborn pups.[38]

Beneficial effects on fertility probably arise from the normalizing and anabolic effects of *Panax ginseng* and *Eleutherococcus*, which serve to rebuild and maintain the health of the endocrine glands. The endocrine glands secrete the hormones that control the reproductive function, and augmenting hormonal secretion could well overcome certain minor causes of infertility.

Composition of *Panax Ginseng* and *Eleutherococcus*

Scientists have identified the active principles of both adaptogens. *Panax ginseng* contains six individual glycosides, called panaxosides *A, B, C, D, E,* and *F.* (A glycoside is a natural plant compound containing a carbohydrate molecule—a sugar—combined with a genin—either an alcohol or a phenol.) Panaxosides *A, B,* and *C* are similar; they contain little sugar and on hydrolysis yield the genin panaxatriol. Panaxosides *D, E,* and *F* contain more sugar and yield the genin panaxadiol. Ginseng also contains variable amounts of simple sugars and other carbohydrates, amino acids, organic acids, fatty acids, sterols, flavonoids, and vitamins including pantothenic acid, biotin, vitamin B-12, thiamine, and riboflavin.

Eleutherococcus also contains six individual glycosides, called eleutherosides *A, B, C, D, E,* and *F.* Eleutherosides *B, D,* and *E* contain syringaresinol. Eleutheroside *A* is daukosterin, and eleutheroside *C* is a galactoside; the structure of eleutheroside *F* is not yet known.[39]

It is possible to separate the glycosides of *Panax ginseng* or *Eleutherococcus* and compare their potency. Pharmacological studies show that some components of each adaptogen exert higher levels of stimulation than others. Much investigation will have to be done before scientists understand how the glycosides interact to work their magic. Nevertheless, it does appear that the whole complex of each plant is more effective than any isolated fraction. If the evidence in favor of the ginsengs continues to mount, science no doubt will search for a way to synthesize adaptogenic compounds.

The Outlook

We have seen that both Siberian and Asiatic ginseng show promise for treatment of a great many disease processes. All the beneficial effects of these adaptogens probably are traceable to their stress-resistant, stimulant, anabolic, normalizing, antioxidant, and antiradical properties. Their almost total lack of side effects makes them attractive for medical use in a broad spectrum of therapies. Certainly *Panax ginseng* and *Eleutherococcus* are valuable for strengthening healthy persons against stress of all kinds and for promoting full and rapid recovery in convalescents. Brekhman tells us that both adaptogens are recommended in Soviet medicine for the following conditions:

- Functional nervous and psychic disorders, such as neuroses, vegetative dystonia, asthenic conditions, climacteric neuroses, and hypochondriacal states.
- Cardiovascular diseases including atherosclerosis, hypotension, and rheumatic heart disease.
- Diabetes.
- Overfatigue, emaciation, convalescence, and postoperative recovery.[40]

In addition, research continues into the potential value of these adaptogens against cancer and other diseases, sterility, and the aging process.

Dr. Norman R. Farnsworth, professor of pharmacognosy, and Dr. John P. Bederka, associate professor of pharmacology, both at the College of Pharmacy at the University of Illinois at the Medical Center in Chicago, recently produced a "critical review on the published works on ginseng." Their conclusions summarize the benefits of *Panax ginseng*, but reflect the natural caution of the responsible investigator and point to the need for further study of adaptogen action:

> The use of ginseng as a general body tonic would seem to be well founded. This impression is based on the described beneficial effects of ginseng regarding cell and tissue growth, physical activities such as swimming and running, and muscular efficiency. This general effect also indicates that ginseng could be an aid to postoperative recovery. The hypoglycemic effect of ginseng would suggest contraindications in patients who are also receiving other hypoglycemic agents. A strict regimen for ginseng is not generally followed and it may be taken as infrequently as once every two weeks. Likewise, ginseng should be used with caution in combination with other drugs that stimulate the central nervous system.
>
> What should not be expected from the use of ginseng? No definite studies are available concerning the effects of ginseng in combating the common cold, and no published evidence has been found concerning the effective use of ginseng as an aphrodisiac in humans. To date, the

use of ginseng seems to involve no more habitua-
tion liability than regular eating. Ginseng has no
apparent utility in diseases caused by bacteria,
parasites, or viruses.

At the present stage of development in the
therapeutic and pharmacologic assessment of ginseng ... well controlled studies with defined ginseng preparations would be a real contribution to
the drug information gap between the East and
the West. Some of the ginseng story is fantasy
and fiction, but much is fact. Ginseng is a plant
that has escaped the eye of the American scientist, who might well benefit by turning his efforts
in this direction.[41]

It appears that the action of *Eleutherococcus* is
stronger than that of *Panax ginseng,* and therefore research probably will be concentrated on *Eleutherococcus.* Nevertheless, the miracles worked by Asiatic
ginseng were the clues that led science to search for
Eleutherococcus, and modern science once again
stands indebted to the herbal wisdom of the barefoot
doctors of the East.

7

Bringing Up Ginseng

THE HARDEST THING about growing ginseng is to resist
pulling up the roots to see who they look like. This
natural urge and the six years of tender loving care
demanded by each plant suggest that the term "nur-
seryman" was coined to describe a ginseng grower.

Bringing up ginseng takes a strong back and the
emotional constitution of an English nanny—but the

benefits certainly justify the effort. Depending on your outlook, it's like cultivating health or growing dollars. The current market puts cured, cultivated ginseng at more than forty dollars a pound; on the other hand, hoarding your crop for personal use will compound its value in terms of your own vitality and longevity.

Ginseng is among the wildest of nature's children and does not take kindly to efforts to tame it. Decades of trial and effort have proved that the route to success lies in duplicating the natural habitat of the plant, rather than in "domesticating" it through the usual cropping methods.

Natural Habitat

In the wild, ginseng is a succulent-rooted herbaceous plant that thrusts up through the leaf-mold soil in shady but well-drained hardwood forest locations, usually on slopes where oak, hickory, beech, maple, basswood, and similar trees abound. The towering trees provide ample shade, but also suck huge quantities of nutrients from the soil, leaving little to nourish the little ginseng shrub. Though the trees shield the ginseng from direct sun, they spread their branches high overhead, allowing the lower growth sufficient indirect light and freely circulating air. The soil is moist but not damp, rather light in texture because of its high content of rotted leaves, and made porous by the probing root systems of the larger forest plants. Ginseng does not flourish near stagnant water, but it may thrive on well-drained slopes bordering a lively stream.

Appearance

Ginseng is very deliberate in its growth, taking five to seven years to mature. All that time the plant is

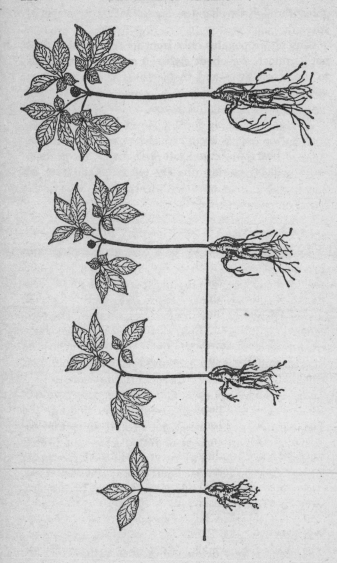

going through its changes, consolidating its essential strength.

Ginseng propagates only from its seed, which does not germinate for about eighteen months after it falls to the forest floor—and then only if it has remained sufficiently moist. In the wild, seeds drop in autumn, but no sturdy sprouts emerge until the second spring following. Then early in May the green stem pushes through the humus layer to stand two to three inches high; it bears one composite leaf made up of three ovate leaflets growing directly out from the apex of the stem. The food energy produced by this first leaf becomes consolidated in the rootstalk, or bud, which will produce the following year's stem and leaves. The plant produces no flowers or fruit during its first year; the first cold snap in autumn will cause the stem to die and break from the rootstalk, leaving the single root bud behind.

The next year the root bud sends up a stem four or five inches high; directly from the apex extend the petioles (stalks) of the two or three compound leaves, each with three or five leaflets. Again the stem dies without producing fruit and leaves a root bud behind.

The third year the stem rises six to nine inches high and bears at its apex three compound leaves, each with five leaflets. From the point where the leafstalks converge on the stem (the apex) a flower stalk grows straight up and produces a small cluster of pale green or yellow-green blossoms. Each blossom develops into a pea-sized green berry; fifteen to fifty berries may be borne on a single ginseng plant. The berries ripen and turn crimson in the fall, when they are favored by birds and squirrels. Each berry contains one, two, or three small flat wrinkled seeds—surely every bit as magic as Jack's beans.

In the spring of the fourth year—and every year thereafter—the ginseng stem shoots up perhaps twelve to twenty inches high and is the thickness of a common pencil. It usually bears four leaves of five leaflets each, and produces a well-formed cluster of berries in the center (see drawing on opposite page). Each year the shrubby parts die back, leaving another little bud on the rootstalk. A. R. Harding whimsically observed,

> Ginseng is very wise and knows its own age. This age the plant shows in two ways. First, by the style of the foliage which changes each year until it is four years old. Second, the age can be determined by counting the scars on the neck of the bud-stem. Each year the stalk . . . goes down, leaving a scar on the neck or perennial root from which it grew. A new bud forms opposite and a little above the old one each year. Counting these stalk scars will give the age of the plant.[1]

The Chinese also made this observation—and cleverly put it to use by sometimes tying silken threads about the rootstalk while it was being treated for market. When the threads were removed, the root looked a few years older, and thus more valuable.

The root is connected to the stem by the slender rootstalk, scarred with the breakoff marks of each year's old stem. The rootstalk has no commerical value, but may be left intact on the root proper as proof of its age. It is said that rootstalks with more than fifty real year-marks are on display in China.

The root itself is fleshy and spindle-shaped, about one-fourth of an inch to an inch in diameter at the thickest part, and from three to eight inches long. Its shape and pale yellow or cream color resemble a young parsnip, but the ginseng root is more deeply marked with cylindrical wrinkles. The size of the root seems to depend more on nutrition and care in cultivation than on age. The root may have one to four or more smaller branches—the "arms" and "legs" that give the root its fancied resemblance to the human form. Cultivated roots don't seem to develop limbs as readily as the wild ones do—which is probably why the wild ginseng is worth almost twice as much on the Asian market.

Figuring the Odds

"Ginseng is truly and wholly a savage. We can no more tame it than we can the partridge."[2] Thus forewarned, the prospective ginseng grower who sets about to mimic ginseng's natural habitat has at least an even chance of success. But you can't fool Mother Nature even part of the time. There are no shortcuts to a bountiful ginseng crop; most of the work must be done by hand on a plant-by-plant basis; and an act of the gods can wipe out the entire plantation after years of effort.

The blandishments of the seed sellers are enticing: "$50,000 yearly per acre possible!" "Huge profits from tiny investment!" No doubt these advertisements are based on fact, but the "tiny investment" refers only to the money paid for seed and doesn't take into account the time, the muscle power, and the potential heartache that are involved. And that $50,000 is decidedly top dollar. Based on a market price of $40 a pound, $50,000 means 1,250 pounds of salable *dried* roots per acre (not counting costs). And *that* translates into about 10,000 to 20,000 healthy ginseng plants that outlast weather, pests, diseases, and your amateurism for at least six years. Furthermore, the lure of $50,000 has to keep your juices up for six to seven years with no income at all from your ginseng crop.

If you're still interested, you must have figured out the angle: After the first crop is harvested, *if* you have established an effective staggering system *and* conquered all the problems of ginseng culture, you just might find yourself in Fat City. And if you are of a peculiar bent, all those little "man roots" might make very groovy child substitutes.

Getting Started

Ginseng seeds are available by mail from several sources, and at varying prices that don't resemble prices for garden variety *anything*. But cheap enough, considering the potential gain. Check the Yellow Pages of your phonebook under "Ginseng" and "Herbs," or try the addresses given in Chapter 8. Write to a few and order from the company that inspires the most confidence. North American companies no doubt sell only seeds of the species *Panax quinquefolium*, which makes sense. Count on about 500 viable seeds per ounce.

Some of the same companies, and others, also sell one-and two-year roots for replanting. They are considerably more expensive than seed, and the buyer runs the risk of introducing disease to his seed crop. In addition, chances are that transplanted roots will never be as strong as those that keep their arms and legs in the ground. In this already high-risk enterprise, seeds would seem to be a safer investment.

At least one company listed in Chapter 8 advertises "live ginseng plants" for a few dollars apiece. A nice idea for an apartment dweller, these plants come with complete care-and-feeding instructions. It's unlikely that one could grow enough plants indoors to satisfy a galloping ginseng regimen, but if you're into talking to plants you could give it a name, and who knows where things might lead?

To start from seed, *act now*. After the seed arrives at your door, you have at least eighteen months to get everything else together while your seed germinates. During that eighteen months, however, the seed must be allowed to work its miracle. Bury it all, spaced well, in a box containing a few inches of the same kind of earth the roots will be transplanted to (see below). Keep the box indoors in a cool, dark place and keep the soil moist, but never damp. Don't allow the seeds to dry out, and don't start the seed until eighteen months before you plan to plant it. If you embark on a different trip meanwhile, give the seeds to a friend.

W. T. Macoun suggests another method of germination:

> The best plan is to stratify the seed as soon as it is ripe, leaving the pulp on. A mixture of sand, loamy soil, and leaf mould is rubbed very fine, so fine that it may be sifted out when desired and leave the seeds. A box with a lid is useful for the storing of the seeds. After putting in about one inch of the prepared soil scatter the seeds thinly on top. Put in half an inch more soil, and so on until all the seeds are in. The box is now closed and buried four or five inches deep in well-drained soil where water will not lie at any time. The seed is left buried for a year. It is taken up the autumn after being buried and sown at once in a bed specially prepared for it, about four feet wide being a convenient size. It should be inclosed by six inch boards for greater protection. The seed bed should be made of soil with a large amount of vegetable matter or leaf

mould in it, of such a character that it will not bake, and free of sticks and stones which might interfere with the development of the roots. The seed is sown about one inch deep, two inches apart, in rows about three inches apart. After seeding, the bed should be mulched for winter with about two inches of decayed leaves. Early in spring remove most of the leaves, the finer parts being left for a mulch on the surface of the soil, through which the young plants will soon make their appearance.[3]

Canopies

Remember ginseng's natural leafy bower and choose a location in which you can provide enough shade. A hillside facing south is the worst possible choice, and an open area of natural woodland is probably best. No doubt you will wish to compromise by erecting an artificial shade system. The canopy may be a framework covered with burlap, a trellis overgrown with vines, or a shade made of lath strips. Whatever the choice, the shade system should cut light intensity by three-fourths with protection concentrated on the top, south, and west exposures. The plants should still receive good indirect light and ventilation. It may be necessary to block out even more light in southern latitudes. Both Stockberger and Harding give more specific instructions for constructing a shading apparatus, as does the U.S. Department of Agriculture's Bulletin 2201, *Growing Ginseng* (price, five cents). Whatever the method, be certain to allow enough room for walking under the canopy.

Making the Bed

Prepare the ginseng bed during the autumn before the spring in which the seed will be planted. Any good garden loam will do for a base; fertilize it with woods earth, rotted leaves, or fine raw bone meal. Lighten the soil with sand if it seems heavy. Ginseng will not thrive in overly rich soil; Rodale's *Encyclopedia of Organic Gardening* recommends an application of bone meal at the rate of one pound per square yard. It is essential that the soil be light enough to drain quickly after a spring rain, but heavy enough to retain sufficient moisture and not harden around the roots.[4]

Drainage of soil is enhanced by a natural sloping of the field. However, ginseng is very persnickety about not having wet feet, and most growers recommend installing clay or concrete drainage tiles two or three feet deep beneath the ginseng beds. This step may sound like an enormous hassle, but if you've promised yourself a ginseng garden, go back to the Yellow Pages and get it over with. Fortunately, installing drainage tiles is a one-shot job.

Plant the germinated seed as soon as the soil can be easily worked in the spring. Work the soil about a foot deep to encourage shapely root development. Set the seeds eight inches apart each way, covered two inches deep.

Biding Your Time

The hard part is accomplished, and you can take up a new hobby or run for senator while waiting for the crop to mature. If the job has been done well, your ginseng bed won't demand constant attention. Cultivate regularly to keep out all signs of weedy or grassy invasion. Stir up the topsoil now and then if it seems cakey. Water if the soil becomes very dry, but take care not to create a swamp.

And by all means *mulch*. Duplication of the autumn leaf fall in a deciduous forest is absolutely essential to making ginseng feel at home. Leaves are best. Other loose mulching material may be used, provided it is free of seeds that will attract mice. Mice are very fond of ginseng roots; if you don't keep them out of the ginseng bed, you'll have two problems—a failing crop and lots of healthy, oversexed, and very together mice.

Apply mulch just before the first frost. Four or five inches of leaves is recommended in cold climates. Remove the mulch in the spring before the ginseng shoots are awake, and then leave the bed alone until the stems are fairly sturdy. If you *must* fertilize to satisfy some basic nurturing instinct, work in a little leaf compost or bone meal, but do so sparingly. The ginseng plant is not a gourmand.

When the flower cluster appears on each plant, cut it off if you wish to encourage root growth. Consider letting a few three- or four-year plants go to seed to supply your next ginseng venture. Or perhaps let the whole bed go to seed, gather the berries, dry them, and collect the seed for sale to another ginseng buff. Producing seed certainly doesn't damage the roots, but they won't grow as fast because part of the plant's energy is siphoned off by the seed production.

Safeguarding the Crop

Moles, mice, and the neighborhood menagerie must be discouraged from using your investment as a lunch bar. Fence off the plantation area to keep out dogs and stray burros. In the face of other scourges, follow whatever course of action suits your situation, but honor the inherent wildness of the ginseng plant and choose organic methods. Chemicals can only adulterate the tonic properties of the root and may kill off more plants than they save.

Ginseng is susceptible to a dreadful assortment of fungus-caused blights, wilts, and rots. All are encouraged by poor drainage, insufficient ventilation, excessive fertilization, and overcrowding. Proper cultural methods will go a long way to prevent troublesome diseases from gaining a foothold. If your crop does fall victim to a fungal disease, you can let the affected plants die in organic splendor or resort to a fungicide such as Bordeaux mixture. Either way the guilt factor is enormous. The references listed in the Bibliography that deal with ginseng ailments will help you choose your method of attack.

Nematodes, also known as eelworms, are fond of most root plants, and ginseng is no exception. These parasitic pests feed on the ginseng root, lay their eggs inside it, and generally make themselves at home. An invasion of these minute worms in full force will cause your ginseng plants to lose a lot of nourishment from their roots, and they may weaken and die. If the leaves of your ginseng plants begin to yellow, and the plants appear to lack vigor, nematodes may be the culprits.

Should you ever suspect that fungi or nematodes have set up housekeeping in your plantation, get in touch with a federal or state agricultural office and explain the problem. Someone there will tell you where to send a soil or plant sample for testing. Once your problem has a name, it's easier to counteract.

The Harvest

During the sixth year of growth, decide whether to harvest or wait one or more years before pulling the roots from the ground. Roots under four inches in length are not desirable for market, and roots of less than six years in age will not have developed the characteristic texture demanded by the Asian buyers.

Though cultivated roots grow faster than wild ones and may exceed four inches early on, they cannot achieve quality before six years has passed. When a root of good quality is broken, it exhibits a typical "soft and waxy fracture."[5]

Careful handling will ensure the value of your crop. If you plan to sell the ginseng, follow the instructions of the company that will buy your crop. Otherwise, begin the harvest in mid-October. Loosen the soil around each plant, working very gently with a trowel. Grasp the plant firmly and draw it from the earth with the utmost care. The object of course is to leave all the little limbs attached to the main body of the root. You may find it easier to dig up the entire root ball with a spade and shake the root free; be certain to dig deep enough and far enough from the root to avoid snapping off the limbs. Shake and gently brush away the soil clinging to the root. Any roots that are not large enough to be "keepers" should be replanted on the spot.

Break the stem from each root and discard it, but try to leave the scarred rootstalk intact on the root. Pile the roots in a cool, dry place and leave them alone for about twenty-four hours. Then wash the roots by spraying or sloshing gently in a pail of water—no soap, no soaking, no scrubbing allowed. The "dirty" color of the root skin is desirable, as it makes the cultivated root more nearly resemble the wild ginseng.

Unless your buyer decrees otherwise, the roots must now be cured before shipping. Place them in a mesh box or basket so that air can circulate freely around each root, thus preventing root rot. The roots should be dried in a heated room, starting with a temperature of 100°F until the roots are wilted and then reducing the temperature to about 80° to 90°F. Allow the roots to dry for four or five weeks, turning them occasionally. The object is described by Harding:

> The essentials of good drying are to start the root so it begins to dry before it sours and after that to dry very slow. If a root is dried fast, the outer shell becomes dry and set or firmly fixed before the inside dries and so forms a shell on the outside that is hard and smooth, but if at least a month is given for drying, the inside of the root dries and as it shrinks, draws the outer shell with it and leaves the skin more wrinkled than if dried quick; and again, in rapid drying the center will show some color instead of breaking white. When it breaks it will break like a piece of glass, where if dried slow, as it should be, the act of breaking will be soft and yielding instead of a snap.[6]

When the roots have dried thoroughly, pull off the tiny root fibers—save them for making tea or extract. The drying process will have reduced the weight of the crop by at least two-thirds. Store the roots in a dark, dust-free place away from all possible contact with moisture. If the roots are exposed to dampness, they will soak up moisture like a sponge and have to be dried again to prevent rot and the formation of mold.

Hawking Your Wares

In any enterprise where West meets East, there are bound to be problems arising from the cultural gap and language difficulties. The ginseng market between North America and China has been operating for more than two centuries. Certain customs have become established, violations of which will only decrease the price fetched by your crop. From time to time ginseng growers try to deceive ginseng buyers, bringing the American product a bad reputation. Once there was an outbreak of ginseng stuffing—hollowing out the core of the root and filling it with iron or lead to increase the weight of the root. Choose a reliable dealer of experience and play fair with him; in turn he will obtain the best possible price your crop can bring in the Asian market.

The Asian buyers are not easily fooled in their quest for ginseng of quality; only by following the time-honored processes outlined above will you produce ginseng adequate to the test. The admonishment of W. W. Stockberger in 1921 holds true today:

> ... growers should strive for quality of product and not for quantity of production, as has been the all too common practice in the past. There is always a ready sale for the cultivated roots which closely resemble the wild in quality and condition, and prudent growers will not fail to adopt the wild root as the standard of future production. The elimination of the poorer grades of cultivated American ginseng ... would tend to insure more uniform prices for the root and to lessen the danger of depressing the market through overproduction.[7]

In days past the amount of land harvested of a ginseng crop in the United States hovered around 150 acres a year. But the market for American ginseng is bound to increase as people the world over become aware of the medicinal value of the herb, and a flourishing market will absorb any quantity of quality ginseng. The results of scientific experimentation have shown that the American species is not chemically inferior to Asian ginseng, and that the cultivated root contains the same properties as the wild root does. As these facts become better known, the superstitious preference for the wild product will wane, and the market for the cultivated ginseng will burgeon.

8

The Root Seller

THE MOST EXCITING WAY to get to the roots is to follow in the footsteps of the hoary seng hunter. There's ginseng in them thar hills, if you live east of the Mississippi. Old timers may bemoan the demise of wild American ginseng, but the fact remains that several million dollars worth of *Panax quinquefolium* finds its way to the Asian market each year. Ralph O. Slenker, a representative of United Fur Brokers in New York and the son of an Ohio seng digger and grower, reports that United Fur alone sells from 30,000 to 45,000 pounds of *wild* ginseng each year at a price that currently hovers around $85 a pound. United Fur buys wild ginseng from seng collectors in the Appalachians and west to Illinois, Missouri, and Wisconsin and sells directly to buyers in Hong Kong and Singapore. Ginseng is a sideline business for United Fur, and there are several other companies in New York alone that deal primarily in ginseng. A lot of wild ginseng must still huddle in the little patches on the forest floor in order to support such a large volume of trade.

Seng hunting has virtues that transcend the medicinal magic of the quarry. It gives purpose to a quiet amble in the woods. Better yet, the quest may lead one into woodlands previously unexplored. Examining leafy shrubs in the hope of finding ginseng will familiarize the hunter with plants he has never noticed before. So a ginseng hunt need never be a complete failure, especially if it is combined with foraging for other herbs.

Should you stumble upon ginseng in the wild, respect it. Dig up only plants that bear four or more leaves of five leaflets each, to be sure the plant is old enough to be of value. Uproot the plant with the utmost care; if the root is not four inches long, replant the whole shrub tenderly in its original hole. Never collect a ginseng plant that has not ripened its seed, which usually happens after September. Finally, be sure to plant the berries of any roots you do take, to ensure replenishment of the ginseng bed.

The Price of Health

If you are convinced of the beneficial nature of Asiatic and Siberian ginseng, you probably will want to experiment with several ways of taking either product. Your final choice will depend largely on the strength of your conviction measured against the size of your purse. Ginseng is expensive, and the best grades are exorbitant. The Japanese have a proverb that warns, "After ginseng, death by hanging." The saying refers to the old Japanese method of punishing debtors (not to the indestructibility of the ginseng user, as I at first supposed).

Nevertheless, health food stores in the United States and Canada report brisk sales of ginseng products. Though the products are expensive, really advanced indulgence in good ginseng will cost one person no more than ten dollars a month. Weighed against the cost of harmful things such as cigarettes and liquor, ginseng comes out as a considerable bargain.

Prices of ginseng vary according to source, but vary

little within categories of sources. Thus health food stores are likely to charge more than mail order houses, which in turn tend to charge more than Oriental drugstores and grocers. Each of these three categories of sources has its advantages. In a health food store you can weigh the value of various products, handle them, read the instructions, and talk with the proprietor—and you can get started on ginseng *today*. Mail order houses provide a larger range of products than most health food stores are willing to stock; some offer discounts for bulk buying and most will send you information on ginseng and their catalogs of herb products on request. Oriental pharmacies are a very good trip all by themselves. If there is one in your area, don't fail to check it out. These drugstores provide endless fascination with their displays of roots, barks, seeds, and herbs of all descriptions and many more mysterious objects, like the velvety deer horns called *panti*. The variety of ginseng products at the Chinese drugstores in New York is astonishing—several brands each of concentrated extracts from China and Korea, teas and extracts of various potencies from Korea, and roots from America, China, and Korea. In the vigorous atmosphere of almost any Oriental grocery store you can purchase ginseng tea and perhaps more concentrated products.

In light of the scientific findings discussed in Chapter 6 it is not unreasonable to predict that the American medical establishment may some day endorse ginseng and other adaptogens. Acupuncture was declared tax-deductible by the U.S. Internal Revenue Service in January 1973. Can ginseng be far behind?

Asiatic Ginseng Roots

Ginseng is sold in the United States and Canada in a wide variety of forms, from instant teas to whole roots. The harvesting and processing of Korean and Chinese ginseng is done entirely under government supervision; the seal on packaged products from these countries at least ensures the identity of the contents. Korean ginseng is widely available. It comes from South Korea, but is gathered in the same mountainous regions as North Korean ginseng. Chinese ginseng from mainland China has recently been allowed into the United States; all Oriental drugstores carry it, and it is gradually turning up in health food stores. American ginseng may be hard to come by except through the mail-order sources listed at the end of this chapter.

Whole roots are shipped to the United States in boxes weighed in *cattys*; one catty equals 1.33 pounds or 21.33 ounces U.S. weight. The roots are identified by source—China, Korea, America, Japan—by grade, and by weight classification. The weight classification indicates the number of roots per catty; thus lower numbers indicate larger roots and higher numbers indicate smaller roots. Larger roots are most expensive. Oddly enough, the numbers don't correspond to the actual quantity of roots: "fifteen-piece style" means nineteen roots; "forty-piece style" means forty-eight roots, and so on.

Grades are applied to roots from China and Korea. In order of quality and price, the grades are

Grade	1971 Hong Kong Wholesale Price (per catty)
Chinese Wild Imperial	$5,000.00
Korean and Chinese Red	216.50
Korean White	196.50
American Wild	133.30
Japanese and American Cultivated	36.60

Because Hong Kong is a duty-free international port, prices there are probably the lowest obtainable anywhere in the world. Chinese and Korean ginseng roots are further classified for quality as:

Heaven	First class
Earth	Second class
Good or Man	Third class
Tails	Fourth class

Thus a classification of, say, Korean Red as "Heaven 15" means that the ginseng roots are top-quality Korean Red roots of a size averaging slightly less than one ounce each. Tails are usually packed by weight only, not by piece count. Chinese Red ginseng may be classified as extra large, large, regular, and small, rather than by number of roots per catty.

Buying ginseng roots can be very confusing to the initiate, for the differences between grades often appear arbitrary and the seller probably has the upper hand. My only advice to the person who wants to use roots of the highest quality is to be patient and try several sources. A butcher once observed that the best cuts of meat go to the person who can call his butcher by name. If you can establish rapport with a ginseng dealer who has access to the best sources, he will be more likely to play straight with you. You are buying an expensive commodity, and you have every right to demand fair play. Ask him to show you the differences between the various grades of roots, and buy by the ounce until you gain experience. Ginseng roots are somewhat less expensive when bought in quantity; perhaps several people could organize for cooperative buying and thus reduce costs.

There are two ways of using the roots—chewing, and boiling or steeping. To chew, either steam the root for five to ten minutes to soften it until it is sliceable, or break it up with force and hold a small piece in your mouth until it softens. Chew a few pieces a day (about a quarter ounce total). Some smokers report that chewing ginseng helps them reduce their desire for cigarettes.

Extracting the active principles from the roots may be less wasteful than chewing them. Use one ounce of roots to a quart of water and boil slowly until the liquid is reduced by half. Or use half an ounce of root to six cups of water and boil slowly for six hours until one cup of liquid remains. Strain out the solids and take two or three tablespoons of the pale brown liquid before meals. Never allow metal to come in contact with ginseng.

Another method of extracting the essence of the root is to steep it in the alcoholic beverage of your choice. Korean and Russian restaurants sometimes offer vodka-ginseng cocktails. To adulterate a tonic like ginseng with the poison of alcohol seems foolish, but many Oriental and Western people recommend it.

Asiatic Ginseng Products

Ginseng powder is sold loose and in capsules, manufactured by simple pulverization of roots and root fibers—usually Korean White. Powders sealed by government authorities in China and Korea are probably unadulterated. Powdered American ginseng is not generally available. Loose powders are packed in jars along with a spoon and dosage directions. Capsules contain from five to ten grains each; directions usually call for three a day to be taken. Powders may also be sprinkled lightly on foods such as meat or cereals.

Ginseng extracts are of two kinds—the highly concentrated "extractum" from China or Korea, sold in small bottles, and the less concentrated Korean extract or elixir, sold in eight-ounce bottles, often containing honey, rice wine, ginseng extract, and a piece of root. The specified dosage of concentrate, in drops, is to be taken in warm water once or twice daily. The weaker elixirs are taken by teaspoonfuls. Extracts are a lovely dark brown color, and the taste is an odd combination of bitter and sweet.

The weakest form of ginseng is instant ginseng or ginseng tea, sold in premeasured packets, in tea bags, or loose in jars. These products are actually granules of processed ginseng. They are taken in hot water and have a weak flavor not unlike mild watercress (however, people accustomed to tobacco and alcohol are likely to describe the taste of ginseng as "dishwater"). Instant ginseng may be made mostly from root fibrils and leaves; rarely is it as strongly tonic as other forms of ginseng. It may be sweetened with sugar or honey.

Other ginseng products include combinations such as Mu Tea, candy bars, and tablets. Recently a line of ginseng cosmetic creams has appeared on the market, presumably intended to capitalize on the rejuvenant properties ascribed to ginseng. To my knowledge, science has produced no evidence that ginseng is absorbed by the external skin or is beneficial to it in any way. Ginseng does have a beneficial effect on living cells, but the outer layers of the skin are made up only of dead, horny, keratinized cells.

Siberian Ginseng

Eleutherococcus products are imported from the USSR only. The roots are not sold whole, probably because the entire plant contains the characteristic medicinal essence, and because there is no mystique attached to any one part of this newly discovered herb—like every good Russian, it works for the good of the people.

Siberian ginseng is available as an extract called "Vigo-Root," a product described in advertisements as "a nontransparent liquid of dark-brown color with specific slightly burning taste and a characteristic odor." The recommended dosage—in drops—is taken in warm water. The only other *Eleutherococcus* product currently available is canned juice containing Siberian ginseng, packaged in single-serving pop-top cans.

WHERE TO BUY ASIATIC AND AMERICAN GINSENG

These sellers of ginseng and other herb products all sell by mail and provide catalogs of their merchandise. Many also maintain retail shops.

Afar East Import/Export Sales
 P.O. Box 9531, North Hollywood, California 91609
 • Powdered Korean ginseng, tea bags, roots.

Aphrodisia
 28 Carmine Street, New York, New York 10014
 • Sells a wide range of Korean ginseng products.

Dominion Herb Distributors, Inc.
 61 St. Catherine Street West, Montreal 129, Quebec
 • Canadian-grown ginseng root.

East Earth Herbs
 Box 181, Route 3, Reedsport, Ontario • Chinese ginseng products.

Essene
 58th and Grays Avenue, Philadelphia, Pennsylvania 19143 • American wild ginseng.

Fmali
 Santa Cruz, California • Sells ginseng from Korea, China, Japan, and U.S.A.

Harmony Foods
191 Freston Road, London, W. 10, England • Sells wild American ginseng and other products.

Heise's Wausau Farms
Route 2, Wausau, Wisconsin 54401 • Home-grown American ginseng, raised and processed at Heise's, whole roots, capsules, and powdered ginseng available.

The Herb Lady
Box 26515, Edendale Station, Los Angeles, California 90026 • Korean ginseng powder, capsules, extract, and Korean White roots; Mu Tea with extra ginseng added.

Indiana Botanic Gardens
Hammond, Indiana 46325 • American wild ginseng.

The Infinity Foods Co.
173 Duane Street, New York, New York 10013 • American wild ginseng.

Jane O'Brien
7 Woodside Drive, Rathfarnum, Dublin, Ireland • Wild American roots when available.

Kiehl's Pharmacy
109 Third Avenue, New York, New York 10003 • A marvelous old-time chemist shop that stocks Korean ginseng extracts, teas, and capsules.

Living Herbs, Inc. (formerly Herb Products Company), 11012 Magnolia Boulevard, North Hollywood, California 91601 • Carries American and Korean roots, as available, at the prevailing market price; capsules of 100 percent pure ground Korean ginseng powder; loose powder or pieces of root of Korean Red and White ginseng.

Nature's Herb Company
281 Ellis Street, San Francisco, California • Ginseng

root powder; the catalog from this company is more interesting than most.

New Pacific Products Company
4064 Marchena Drive, Los Angeles, California 90065 • Full line of Korean ginseng—tea bags, tea powder, liquid, capsules, bulk powder, concentrated extract, Red and White roots, and Korean ginseng candy ("widely used by U.S. 8th Army in Korea").

Nichol's Garden Nursery
1190 North Pacific Highway, Albany, Oregon 97321 • Ginseng tea; marvelous catalog on request.

Palomar Herbs
105 Hudson Street, New York, New York 10013 • Sells capsules, Korean Red and White (heaven) roots, concentrate, and tea bags.

Return Co.
Box 373, Woodstock, New York 12498 • Wild American ginseng roots, unprocessed.

Superior Trading Company
867 Washington Street, San Francisco, California 94108 • Complete line of Korean ginseng products—concentrate, extract, granules, powder, tea bags; Chinese Red roots available.

Westward Products Co.
P.O. Box 1032, Studio City, California 91604 • Korean ginseng capsules and powder.

World-Wide Herbs, Ltd.
11 St. Catherine Street East, Montreal 129, Quebec • Korean ginseng, whole, powdered, and in tablets and sachets (packets of instant ginseng).

WHERE TO BUY SIBERIAN GINSENG

Eleutherococcus is not widely available in the United States except by mail order. Try these firms:

Afar East Import/Export Sales
P.O. Box 9531, North Hollywood, California 91609
• Siberian ginseng extract ("Vigo-Root").

Frozen Natural Foods, Inc.
1055 Shafter Street, San Diego, California 92106
• Carries Siberian ginseng extract (50-day supply)
and extract mixed with juice in single-serving pop-
top cans ("Siberian Ginseng Apricot Nectar").

The Herb Lady
Box 26515, Edendale Station, Los Angeles, Cali-
fornia 90026 • Siberian ginseng extract ("Vigo-
Root").

Imedex International
1055 Shafter Street, San Diego, California, 92106
• Exclusive distribution rights to *Eleutherococcus* in
the Western Hemisphere.

Westward Products Co.
P.O. Box 1032, Studio City, California, 91604
• Siberian ginseng extract ("Vigo-Root").

CONTACTS FOR GROWERS

Panax ginseng seeds, plants, and roots are available
from several suppliers:

Black Forest Botanicals
Box 34 F, Yuba, Wisconsin 54672 • Seeds and plants.

F. B. Collins
Viola, Iowa 52350 • Seeds and roots.

Ginseng Gardens
Asheville, North Carolina 28801 • Seeds and plants.

Glass' Ginseng Exchange
Box 336, Rochdale Station, Jamaica, New York 11434
• Buys ginseng crops and sells seeds and information. This firm gives out no free information and
asks $2 for a seed sample and instructions.

J. V. Hardacre
Route 1, Wadsworth, Ohio 44281 • Seeds and plants.

Lakeland Nursery Sales
Dept. L-579, Hanover, Pennsylvania 17331 • Live ginseng plants with growing instructions.

Redwood City Seed Company
Box 361, Redwood City, California 94061 • American ginseng plants.

Roots O' Gold
Route 2, Box 74, LeCenter, Minnesota 56057 • Seeds and plants.

Still's Ginseng Mountain
214 RG-4, Echodale, Knoxville, Tennessee 37902 • Supplies seeds and roots to growers.

The following firms deal in ginseng and may be willing to buy your crop. Contact them well in advance to see whose terms suit you best. They may have particular requirements as to the condition in which roots are to be delivered to them, and it is best to find such information out as early as possible.

William J. Boehner & Co.
259 West 30th Street, New York, New York 10001.

Consolidated Fur & Ginseng Co.
157 West 29th Street, New York New York 10001.

Hensely Fur Company
Box 153, Waynesville, Missouri 65583.

F. C. Taylor Fur Company
227 Market Street, Louisville Kentucky 40202.

United Fur Brokers
258 West 29th Street, New York, New York 10001.

Q. C. Plott Fur & Ginseng Company
4062 Peachtree Road, Atlanta, Georgia 30319.

Notes

Chapter 1. *Herbal Wisdom of the Ancients*

1. Edward H. Hume, *The Chinese Way in Medicine* (Baltimore: Johns Hopkins Press, 1940), p. 5.
2. See, for example, Ralph C. Crozier, *Traditional Medicine in Modern China* (Cambridge: Harvard University Press, 1968); and István Pálos, *The Chinese Art of Healing* (New York: Herder and Herder, 1971).
3. Crozier, p. 14.
4. Pálos, pp. 181–82.

Chapter 2. *The Root of Heaven*

1. G. A. Stuart, *Chinese Materia Medica: Vegetable Kingdom* (Shanghai: Presbyterian Mission Press, 1928) p. 298.
2. Martha W. Lear, "Is There a Male Menopause?" *The New York Times Magazine,* 28 January 1973, p. 64.
3. Jeannie Rose, *Herbs & Things* (New York: Grosset & Dunlap, 1972), pp. 60–61.
4. Richard Lucas, *Nature's Medicines* (New York: Parker Publishing Co., 1969), p. 157.
5. Paul M. Kourennoff and George St. George, *Russian Folk Medicine* (New York: Pyramid Publications, 1971), p. 149.
6. Lin Yutang, *My Country and My People* (New York: John Day Company, 1939), p. 152.
7. C. T. Collyer, "The Culture and Preparation of Ginseng in Korea," in *Bulletin of the Royal Asiatic Society, Korean Branch, Seoul* 3, part 1 (1903):30.
8. Stuart, chapters 4 and 5, *passim.*
9. A. Chamfrault and Ung Kang Sam, *Traité de Médecine Chinoise* (Angoulême: Éditions Coquemard, 1961).

10. Sakurazawa Nyoiti, *You Are All Sanpaku* (New York: University Books, 1965), p. 158.

11. Masaru Toguchi, *Oriental Herbal Wisdom* (New York: Pyramid Publications, 1973).

12. Kourennoff and St. George, p. 145.

13. Mrs. M. Grieve, *A Modern Herbal* (New York: Hafner Publishing Co., 1940), 1, p. 356.

Chapter 3.   *Asiatic Ginseng and the Siberian Challenger*

1. Douglas E. McDowell, *Ginseng—Its History, Cultivation, Market Value, and Profits* (privately published, 1902) p. 27.

2. G. A. Stuart, *Chinese Materia Medica: Vegetable Kingdom* (Shanghai: Presbyterian Mission Press, 1928), pp. 301–302.

3. J. F. Shephard, *U.S. Consular Report* 14, no. 46 (1884):228.

4. George C. Foulk, *Foreign Relations of the United States—1885*, pp. 329–330.

5. Nicholas Pike, *Foreign Relations of the United States—1902*, p. 242.

6. William Morse, "Chinese Medicine," *Clio Medica*, vol. 7, p. 24.

7. Henry B. Miller, "Ginseng," *U.S. Consular Report* 75 (1904): p. 497.

8. Euell Gibbons, *Stalking the Healthful Herbs* (New York: David McKay, 1966), p. 161.

9. C. T. Collyer, "The Culture and Preparation of Ginseng in Korea," *Bulletin of the Royal Asiatic Society, Korean Branch, Seoul* 3, part 1 (1903):27.

10. Father Jartoux, "The description of a Tartarian plant, called ginseng; with an account of its virtues (1714)," *Royal Society of London, Philosophical Translations* 28:240.

11. J. M. Canny, "The Sea-Board of Russian Manchuria," *Journal of the North-China Branch of the Royal Asiatic Society* (Shanghai: Presbyterian Mission Press, 1864), pp. 85–86.

12. John Burns, "Canada and China May Trade Doctors," *The New York Times*, 27 April 1973, p. 12.

Chapter 4. *The Ginseng Boom in America*

1. Father Jartoux, "The description of a Tartarian plant, called ginseng; with an account of its virtues (1714)," *Royal Society of London, Philosophical Translations* 28:237–247.

2. Peter Kalm, *En resa til Norra Amerika* [A Journey to North America], 1753.

3. A. R. Harding, *Ginseng and Other Medicinal Plants* (Columbus, Ohio, 1908), p. 43.

4. W. P. Cutler, *The Life, Journals, and Correspondence of Mannasseh Cutler* (1888), 1, p. 402.

5. André Michaux, *Voyage a l'Ouest des Monts Allegheny* (Paris: 1804).

6. Daniel M. Henderson, *Yankee Ships in China Seas* (Freeport, N.Y.: Books for Libraries Press, 1946), p. 46.

7. Virgil Vogel, *American Indian Medicine* (Norman, Okla.: University of Oklahoma Press, 1970), p. 130.

8. *Ibid.*, p. 131.

9. *Ibid.*, p. 99.

10. William Byrd, *The History of the Dividing Line Between Virginia and North Carolina as Run in 1728–29* (Richmond, Va.: 1866), pp. 161–162.

11. Vogel, pp. 309–310.

12. Douglas E. McDowell, *Ginseng—Its History, Cultivation, Market Value, and Profits* (privately published, 1902), p. 21.

Chapter 5. *Drums Along the Seng Trail*

1. Michael A. Weiner, *Earth Medicines—Earth Foods* (New York: The Macmillan Co., 1972), p. 5.

2. W. J. Hoffman, "The Midewiwin of the Ojibwa," in *Seventh Annual Report*, Bureau of American Ethnology, 1885–1886, p. 239.

3. *Ibid.*, pp. 241–242.

4. *Ibid.*, p. 243.

5. Huron H. Smith, "Ethnobotany of the Ojibwa Indians," *Bulletin of the Public Museum of the City of Milwaukee* 4, no. 3 (1932):356–57.

6. Huron H. Smith, "Ethnobotany of the Menomini Indians," *Bulletin of the Public Museum of the City of Milwaukee* 4, no. 1 (1923):24.

7. Huron H. Smith, "Ethnobotany of the Forest Potawat-omi Indians," *Bulletin of the Public Museum of the City of Milwaukee* 7, no. 1 (1932): 41.

8. Huron H. Smith, "Ethnobotany of the Meskwaki Indians," *Bulletin of the Public Museum of the City of Milwaukee* 4, no. 2 (1928):197.

9. *Ibid.*, p. 204.

10. James Mooney, "The Sacred Formulas of the Chero-kee," in *Seventh Annual Report*, Bureau of American Ethnology, 1885–1886, p. 326.

11. John R. Swanton, "Religious Beliefs and Medicinal Practices of the Creek Indians," in *Forty-Second Annual Report*, Bureau of American Ethnology, 1924–1925, p. 656.

12. *Ibid.*, p. 511.

13. *Ibid.*, p. 485.

14. W. M. Beauchamp, "Onandaga Plant Names," *Journal of American Folk-Lore* 15, no. 17 (1902):97–98.

15. Virgil Vogel, *American Indian Medicine* (Norman, Okla: University of Oklahoma Press, 1970), p. 310.

Chapter 6. *The Evidence*

1. I. I. Brekhman and I. V. Dardymov, "New Substances of Plant Origin Which Increase Nonspecific Resis-tance," *Annual Review of Pharmacology* 9 (1969): 421.

2. René Dubos, *Man, Medicine, and Environment* (New York: New American Library, 1968), p. 69.

3. Adelle Davis, *Let's Get Well* (New York: Harcourt, Brace & World, 1965), pp. 16–17.

4. I. I. Brekhman, *Eleuterokokk* [Eleutherococcus] (Leningrad: Izdatel'stvo "Nauka," 1968), p. 8.

5. Brekhman and Dardymov, p. 422.

6. *Ibid.*

7. *Ibid.*, p. 423.

8. *Ibid.*, p. 424.

9. *Ibid.*

10. *Ibid.*

11. Jeannine Swayne, *Los Angeles Herald-Examiner*, 20 February 1972, p. 4.

12. W. Sterner and A. M. Kirchdorfer, "Comparative Performance Tests on Mice with Standard Ginseng Extract and a Ginseng Extract Containing Gerothera-

peutic Preparation," *Zeitschrift für Gerontologie* 3, no. 5 (1970):307–12.

13. Brekhman, p. 5.
14. *Ibid.*
15. K. Tagaki, H. Saito, and M. Tsuchiya, "Pharmacological Studies of *Panax ginseng* Root," *Japanese Journal of Pharmacology* 22, no. 3 (June 1972).
16. Brekhman, p. 6.
17. P. P. Golikov, "The Effect of Ginseng on the Duration of Life in White Mice With Strychnine Poisoning," *Information for a Study of Ginseng and Other Drugs of the Soviet Far East* 7 (1966):279–81.
18. N. V. Lazarev and I. I. Brekhman, "Influence of Preparations of *Eleutherococcus senticosus* on Neoplastic Disease," *Medical Science and Service (India)* 4 (1967):9–13.
19. Brekhman, p. 7.
20. *Ibid.*, p. 13.
21. Tagaki, Saito, and Tsuchiya.
22. Brekhman, p. 11.
23. Norman R. Farnsworth and John P. Bederka, Jr., "Ginseng: Fantasy, Fiction, or Fact?" *Tile and Till* Autumn 1973.
24. *Ibid.*
25. G. N. Bezdetko, *Eleuterokokk i drugie adaptogenie dalnevostochnih rasteniy [Eleutherococcus and other adaptogens from Far Eastern plants]* (Vladivostok: Primorskoe Knizhnoe izdatel'stvo, 1966), pp. 81–84.
26. Brekhman, p. 9.
27. Lazarev and Brekhman, p. 13.
28. Kyung-Dong Lee and Richard P. Huemer, "Antitumoral Activity of *Panax ginseng* Extracts," *Japanese Journal of Pharmacology* 21 (1971):299–302.
29. Brekhman and Dardymov, p. 423.
30. Brekhman, pp. 11, 14, 16.
31. G. A. Vasilev, A. N. Ukshe, and V. I. Sokolov, "Radioprotective Effect of Ginseng Root Extract," *Radiobiologiya* 9, no. 4 (1969):570–73; Brekhman and Dardymov, p. 423.
32. Brekhman, pp. 15–16.
33. *Ibid.*, p. 12.
34. T. L. Bykhovtsova, "Morphological Changes in Rabbit Blood Under the Effect of Ginseng and *Eleutherococcus* Root Preparations," *Izv. Akad. Nauk SSSR*

Ser. Biol. 5 (1971):713–17; Yoon Keun Kim, *Journal of the Catholic Medical College (Seoul)* 18 (1971): 103–112; T. L. Bykhovtsova, "The Effect of Ginseng Preparations and Eleutherococcus Roots on Carbohydrate Metabolism," *Izv. Akad. Nauk SSSR Ser. Biol.* 6 (1970):915–18.

35. G. C. Yuan and Chang R. Shihman, "Compounds That Prolong Postmitotic Life Span of Cultured Human Amnion Cells," *Journal of Gerontology* 24, no. 1 (1969): 82–85; Il Sung Yu, "Effects of Ginseng on Skin Mast Cells in Rats," *Journal of the Catholic Medical College (Seoul)* 15 (1969): 1–11; Jun Won Kang and Il Chun Chung, "Effects of Ginseng Extract on Epithelium in Normal and Stressed Rats," *Journal of the Catholic Medical College (Seoul)* 18 (1970): 1–14; H. Oura et al., "Synthesis and Characterization of Nuclear RNA Induced by Radix Ginseng Extract in Rat Liver," *Chemical and Pharmaceutical Bulletin* 19 (1971): 1598–1605; Chong Soo Chun, "Influence of Ginseng Extract on Lymphoid Tissues," *Journal of the Catholic Medical College (Seoul)* 19 (1970): 317–31; Won Ho Park and Chul Kim, "Effect of Ginseng on Visceral Nucleic Acid Content of Rats," *Journal of the Catholic Medical College (Seoul)* 19 (1970): 83–93; and Soon Yong You, "Effect of Ginseng on ATPase Activity of Mitochondria," *Seoul Journal of Medicine* 12, no. 3 (1971): 173–80.

36. Brekhman and Dardymov, pp. 425–26.

37. Keizo Shida, Jun Shimazaki, and Etsuro Urano, *Japanese Journal of Fertility and Sterility* 15, no. 2 (1970): 113–18.

38. Brekhman, p. 3.

39. I. I. Brekhman and I. V. Dardymov, *Lloydia* 32, no. 1 (1969): 46–51.

40. Brekhman, p. 17.

41. Farnsworth and Bederka, pp. 12.

Chapter 7. *Bringing Up Ginseng*

1. A. R. Harding, *Ginseng and Other Medicinal Plants* (Columbus, Ohio, 1908) p. 59.

2. *Ibid.*, p. 85.

3. W. T. Macoun, "Ginseng Culture," *Pamphlet No. 7*, U.S. Department of Agriculture, 1912, p. 2.

4. J. I. Rodale and staff, *The Encyclopedia of Organic Gardening* (Emmaus, Penn.: Rodale Books, 1970), pp. 430–31.
5. W. W. Stockberger, "Ginseng Culture," *Farmers' Bulletin No. 1184,* U.S. Department of Agriculture, 1921, p. 11.
6. Harding, pp. 122–23.
7. Stockberger, p. 15.

Bibliography

The American Journal of Chinese Medicine. Vol. I, No. 1, published February 1973; subsequent issues to be published quarterly.

Anderson, Donald J. "Wild Ginseng: The Magic Root," *Field & Stream,* February 1971, p. 67.

Bates, W. A. *Ginseng Roots.* Cuba, N. Y.: 1904.

Bowman, N. H. *The History of Korean Medicine.* Seoul: Severance Union Medical College, 1915.

Brekhman, I. I. *Eleuterokokk* [Eleutherococcus]. Leningrad: Izdatel'stvo "Nauka," 1968.

Butz, George C. "Cultivation of American Ginseng in Pennsylvania." Pennsylvania Department of Agriculture, *Bulletin No. 27,* 1897.

Carles, William R. "Report of a Journey from Söul to the Phyöng-kang Gold Washings." *Bulletin of the Great Britain Foreign Office of Corea,* 1885, no. 3.

——. "Report on a Journey in Two Central Provinces of Corea." *Bulletin of the Great Britain Foreign Office of Corea,* 1884, no. 1.

Chakraberty, C. *A Comparative Hindu Materia Medica.* Calcutta, 1923.

Chamfrault, A., and Ung Kang Sam, M. *Traité de Médecine Chinoise.* Angoulême: Éditions Coquemard, 1961.

Coe, Charles H. "Ginseng." *Scientific American Supplement* 57 (1904): 23704–23705.

Collyer, Rev. C. T. "The Culture and Preparation of Ginseng in Korea." *Bulletin of the Royal Asiatic Society, Korean Branch, Seoul.* Vol. 3, part 1, pp. 18–30.

Copeland, Bob. "Herbal Remedies—Next Medical Import from China." *Health Foods and Nutrition News,* Spring 1973, p. 35.

Crozier, Ralph C. *Traditional Medicine in Modern China.* Cambridge: Harvard University Press, 1968.

Culpeper, Nicholas. *The English Physician.* London: 1826.

Federov, I. I. *Otscherki po narodnoj kitajskoi medizine* [A Treatise on Chinese Folk Medicine]. Moscow: Medgiz Press, 1960.

Fujikawa, Yu. "Japanese Medicine," *Clio Medica, A Series of Primers on the History of Medicine*. Vol. 12. New York: P.B. Hoeber, 1934.

Gibbons, Euell. *Stalking the Healthful Herbs*. New York: David McKay Company, 1970.

Grieve, Mrs. M. *A Modern Herbal*. New York: Hafner Publishing Company, 1940.

"Growing Ginseng." U.S. Department of Agriculture, *Bulletin No. 2201*.

Harding, A. R. *Ginseng and Other Medicinal Plants*. Columbus, Ohio, 1908.

Hoffman, W. J. "The Midewiwin of the Ojibwa." *Seventh Annual Report*. Bureau of American Ethnology, 1885–1886, pp. 241–242.

Huard, Pierre, and Wong, Ming. *Chinese Medicine*. Translated by Bernard Fielding. New York: McGraw-Hill Book Co., 1968.

Hume, Edward H. *The Chinese Way in Medicine*. Baltimore: The Johns Hopkins Press, 1940.

Kourennoff, Paul M., and St. George, George. *Russian Folk Medicine*. New York: Pyramid Publications, 1971.

Kreig, Margaret B. *Green Medicine: The Search for Plants That Heal*. Chicago: Rand McNally and Co., 1965.

Krutch, Joseph W. *Herbal*. New York: G. P. Putnam Sons, 1965.

Lafitau, Fr. Joseph. *Memoire . . . concernant la précieux plante du gin-seng*. Montréal: Typographie de Senecal, Daniel et Compagnie, 1858.

Lucas, Richard. *Nature's Medicines*. New York: Parker Publishing Company, 1969.

McDowell, Douglas E. *Ginseng—Its History, Cultivation, Market Value, and Profits*. Privately published, 1902.

Macoun, W. T. "Ginseng Culture." U.S. Department of Agriculture, *Pamphlet No. 7*, 1902.

Meyer, Joseph E. *The Herbalist*. Rev. ed. New York: Sterling, 1968.

Miller, Henry B. "Ginseng." *U.S. Consular Report* 75 (1904): 495–500.

Mooney, James. "The Sacred Formulas of the Cherokees." *Seventh Annual Report*. Bureau of American Ethnology, 1885–1886, pp. 301–397.

Morse, William. "Chinese Medicine." *Clio Medica, A Series of Primers on the History of Medicine.* Vol. 7. New York: P.B. Hoeber, 1934.

Nadkarni, K. *Indian Materia Medica.* Bombay: Popular Book Depot, 1954.

Nyoiti, Sakurazawa. *You Are All Sanpaku.* English version by William Dufty. New York: University Books, 1965.

Pálos, Dr. István. *The Chinese Art of Healing.* New York: Herder and Herder, 1971.

Panton, J. H. "Ginseng." Ontario Agricultural College Experimental Station *Bulletin No. 65,* 1891.

Potter's New Cyclopaedia of Medicinal Herbs and Shrubs. Reedited and enlarged by R. W. Wren. London: Harper & Row, Publishers, 1972.

Read, Bernard E. *Chinese Materia Medica.* Peiping: 1932–1934.

Regnault, J. E. J. *La Médecine et Pharmacie Chez les Chinois et les Annamites.* Paris: 1902.

Rodale, J. I., and staff. *The Encyclopedia of Organic Gardening.* Emmaus, Penn.: Rodale Books, 1970.

Rose, Jeannie. *Herbs & Things.* New York: Grosset & Dunlap, 1972.

Rosenbaum, Joseph. "Phytophthora Disease of Ginseng." *Bulletin 363.* Cornell University Experimental Station of the New York State College of Agriculture. October 1915.

Smith, H. Huron. "Ethnobotany of the Menomini Indians." *Bulletin of the Public Museum of the City of Milwaukee.* Vol. 4, no. 1, 1923.

——. "Ethnobotany of the Meskwaki Indians." *Bulletin of the Public Museum of the City of Milwaukee.* Vol. 4, no. 2, 1928.

——. "Ethnobotany of the Ojibwa Indians." *Bulletin of the Public Museum of the City of Milwaukee.* Vol. 4, no. 3, 1932.

——. "Ethnobotany of the Forest Potawatomi Indians." *Bulletin of the Public Museum of the City of Milwaukee.* Vol. 7, no. 1, 1933.

Special Crops (a magazine concerning the cultivation of ginseng, goldenseal, and other medicinal plants). 1903–1935.

Stockberger, W. W. "Ginseng Culture." U.S. Department of Agriculture, *Farmers' Bulletin No. 1184,* 1921.

Stuart, G. A. *Chinese Materia Medica: Vegetable King-*

dom. A revision of the original work by F. Porter Smith. Shanghai: Presbyterian Mission Press, 1928.

Sun Ju Lee. *Korean Folk Medicine.* Seoul: Seoul National University, 1966.

Swanton, John R. "Religious Beliefs and Medical Practices of the Creek Indians." *Forty-Second Annual Report to the Secretary of the Smithsonian Institute.* Bureau of American Ethnology, 1924–1925.

Taylor, Norman. *Plant Drugs That Changed the World.* New York: Dodd, Mead & Co., 1965.

Vincent, Eugene. *La Médecine en Chine au XXe Siècle.* Paris: G. Steinheil, 1915.

Vogel, Virgil. *American Indian Medicine.* Norman, Okla: University of Oklahoma Press, 1970.

Wallnöfer, Heinrich, and von Rottauscher, Anna. *Chinese Folk Medicine and Acupuncture.* Translated by Marion Palmedo. New York: Bell Publishing Co., 1965.

Weiner, Michael A. *Earth Medicine—Earth Foods.* New York: The Macmillan Company, 1972.

Whetzel, H. H., and Rosenbaum, J. "The Diseases of Ginseng and Their Control." U.S. Department of Agriculture Bureau of Plant Industry, *Bulletin No. 250,* 1922.

Wong, K. *History of Chinese Medicine.* Tientsin, China: The Tientsin Press, Ltd., 1932.

Yutang, Lin. *My Country and My People.* New York: John Day Company, 1939.

Index

are you
missing out on
some great
Pyramid books?

You can have any title in print at
Pyramid delivered right to your door!
To receive your Pyramid Paperback
Catalog, fill in the label below (use a
ball point pen please) and mail to
Pyramid . . .